HOW TO
WIN A
FIGHT

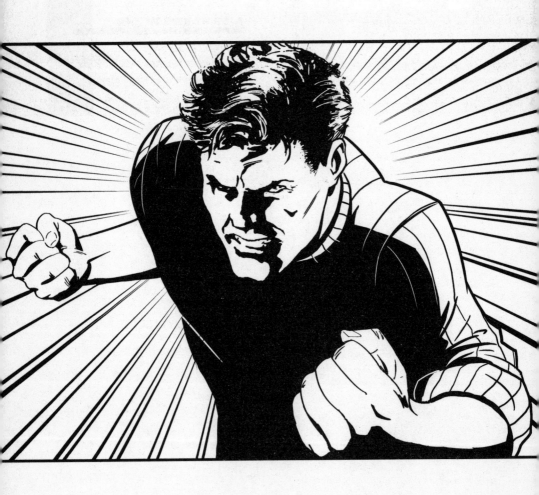

HOW TO WIN A FIGHT

A GUIDE TO AVOIDING AND SURVIVING VIOLENCE

Lawrence Kane
and Kris Wilder

GOTHAM BOOKS

GOTHAM BOOKS
Published by Penguin Group (USA) Inc.
375 Hudson Street, New York, New York 10014, U.S.A.
Penguin Group (Canada), 90 Eglinton Avenue East, Suite 700, Toronto, Ontario
M4P 2Y3, Canada (a division of Pearson Penguin Canada Inc.); Penguin Books Ltd,
80 Strand, London WC2R 0RL, England; Penguin Ireland, 25 St Stephen's Green,
Dublin 2, Ireland (a division of Penguin Books Ltd); Penguin Group (Australia),
250 Camberwell Road, Camberwell, Victoria 3124, Australia (a division of Pearson
Australia Group Pty Ltd); Penguin Books India Pvt Ltd, 11 Community Centre,
Panchsheel Park, New Delhi—110 017, India; Penguin Group (NZ), 67 Apollo Drive,
Rosedale, Auckland 0632, New Zealand (a division of Pearson New Zealand Ltd);
Penguin Books (South Africa) (Pty) Ltd, 24 Sturdee Avenue, Rosebank,
Johannesburg 2196, South Africa

Penguin Books Ltd, Registered Offices: 80 Strand, London WC2R 0RL, England

Published by Gotham Books, a member of Penguin Group (USA) Inc.

First printing, October 2011

10 9 8 7 6 5 4 3 2 1
Copyright © 2011 by Lawrence A. Kane and Kris Wilder

LIBRARY OF CONGRESS CATALOGING-IN-PUBLICATION DATA
Kane, Lawrence A. (Lawrence Alan)
   How to win a fight : a guide to surviving violence / Lawrence Kane and Kris Wilder.
      p.   cm.
   Includes bibliographical references.
   ISBN 978-1-59240-631-9 (pbk.)
   1. Self-defense.   2. Violence—Prevention.   3. Violence—Psychological aspects.
I. Wilder, Kris.   II. Title.
   GV1111.K258   2011
   613.66—dc23   2011025160

Illustrations by Matt Haley

Printed in the United States of America

Set in Olympian Std with Neographik MT and NeoTech Std

Designed by Sabrina Bowers

While the author has made every effort to provide accurate telephone numbers and
Internet addresses at the time of publication, neither the publisher nor the author
assumes any responsibility for errors, or for changes that occur after publication.
Further, the publisher does not have any control over and does not assume any
responsibility for author or third-party Web sites or their content.

For Laura Vanderpool.

Without her, we would be grunting cavemen not knowing if we should eat the paper or write on it.

Contents

WARNING: *Self-defense is legal, but fighting is illegal. If you're not defending yourself, you are fighting—which will send you to jail or worse. Readers are encouraged to be aware of all appropriate local and national laws relating to self-defense, reasonable force, and the use of weaponry, and act in accordance with all applicable laws at all times. Understand that while legal definitions and interpretations are generally uniform, there are small—but very important—differences from state to state. To stay out of jail, you need to know these differences. Neither the authors nor the publisher assumes any responsibility for the use or misuse of information contained in this book.*

Nothing in this document constitutes a legal opinion nor should any of its contents be treated as such. While the authors believe that everything herein is accurate, any questions regarding specific self-defense situations, legal liability, and/or interpretation of federal, state, or local laws should always be addressed by an attorney-at-law. This text relies on public news sources to gather information on various crimes and criminals described herein. While news reports of such incidences are generally accurate, they are on occasion incomplete or incorrect. Consequently, all suspects should be considered innocent until proven guilty in a court of law.

*When it comes to martial arts, self-defense, and related topics, no text, no matter how well written, can substitute for professional, hands-on instruction. These materials should be used **FOR ACADEMIC STUDY ONLY.***

Foreword

by Sergeant Rory Miller

Sergeant Rory Miller is the author of *Meditations on Violence: A Comparison of Martial Arts Training & Real World Violence*, *Violence: A Writer's Guide*, and *Facing Violence: Preparing for the Unexpected*. He has studied martial arts since 1981. He has received college varsities in judo and fencing, and holds *mokuroku* (teaching certificate) in Sosuishitsu-ryu jujutsu. He is a corrections officer and tactical team leader who teaches and designs courses in defensive tactics, close-quarters combat, and use-of-force policy and application for law enforcement and corrections officers. He recently spent a year in Iraq helping the government there develop their prison management system. A veteran of hundreds of violent confrontations, he lectures on realism and training for martial artists and writers.

Kris and Lawrence are nice guys.

They're tough guys, and they have the skill to put a hurtin' on you. They've both spilled blood and smelled it. But they're nice and intelligent and a little naïve—because they think they can convince you that violence is something you want to avoid just using facts.

There are tons of facts in here. Facts and stories, and really good advice. Whatever you paid in money for the book, someone else paid in blood for the lessons. All that advice came at a price.

All of Lawrence's statistics were originally written in some poor bastard's blood on some sidewalk.

Lawrence and Kris think that they can get this through your head with facts and words. I don't think you're that smart.

When they write how hard it will be looking in the mirror every morning knowing that you have killed someone, they know this is true—because every non-sociopath they have talked to tells them how hard it is. Just words. In your adolescent fantasy (and even in your fifties, many of your fantasies are purely adolescent) being a "killer" seems pretty cool.

Let me lay it out as these two fine men tried to lay it out in this little black book: There are tons of things that are cool to think about that suck to do. Some suck so bad that the memory becomes a pain separate from the thing you are remembering.

You will read about heroes in here. Your little eyes will get all shiny and you will think, "I could do that!" And it's a good feeling because in your little Hollywood-influenced world, the hero gets the acclaim of people and the love of a beautiful stranger. In the world of this book, the same hero gets months of physical therapy and torturous surgeries, and "it" (the arm, the knee, the hand, the eye, the back) never, ever works the same way again. Never.

Or maybe it goes another way. Maybe the relatives of the guy who attacked you, though they have been afraid of him for years, come out of the woodwork and get a small army of attorneys and start remembering how he was "a good boy, very caring" or he "was turning his life around." That small army of attorneys will have a mission—to take money from you to give to the family of the person you injured or to the person himself. If a home-invasion robber can sue and win for "loss of earnings," there's very little hope that good intentions will protect you. What seems worse, to me, is that you wind up giving your earnings, your money, and your assets to someone you don't even like, possibly someone with a long history of crime, certainly to someone who doesn't deserve it.

That's the good option, because the boys in blue may show up. You may find some special stainless-steel bling ratcheted over your wrists and get a nice ride to the big building with the laminated

Lexan windows and sometimes real bars for doors. When you hear and feel that cold electronic lock slam shut behind you, you will know that your life has changed forever. Then you might meet me or someone very like me. If you decide to sip twice at the well of violence, it will be my job to stop you, and I will stop you cold. It will hurt quite a lot.

Kris and Lawrence tell good stories about fights and killings that don't happen. A strategist takes the lesson, and they hope, in their naïve and sincere way, that the reader (that's you) wants to be a strategist. I know better. You'll skim those stories and get to the bloody ones, imagining in vivid Technicolor what a knife can do, just like at the movies. But the movies never get the screams quite right, and sometimes the real memories that stay with you are the smells: rotten sh*t and fresh blood and decomposition and the soapy, meaty smell of fresh brains.

Kris and Lawrence are so careful to go over the complexity of the subject. Violence isn't just violence. It happens in a social context, a legal context, and a medical context, and they all play off one another. They put it in your face that you may lose your home, your career, your family, your sight . . . to save a wallet with fourteen dollars or so that some strangers won't think bad thoughts about you. Is it enough for them to put it in your face? Will you read it?

I don't think you're that smart. I don't think you can see past your own ego. I think that you will risk your own life and piss away good information to protect your daydreams.

Maybe not. Prove me wrong. Read the book, read it carefully. Follow the advice, avoid the risks, and become a *strategist*. Prove to me that you are smarter than I think you are.

I won't hold my breath.

Sergeant Rory Miller
www.chirontraining.com
www.chirontraining.blogspot.com

Prologue

At eighteen, I (Andy C) found myself outside an all-ages pool hall in Redmond, Washington. If Redmond sounds familiar to you, it should; it is the home of Microsoft corporate headquarters, the home of programmers, computer geeks, and ninety-eight-pound nerds. I was standing in the heart of suburbia, bleeding badly from my face. The three men who jumped me outside the pool hall started hitting me hard, driving me onto the ground, which was more dirt than gravel. I tried to fight but they had gotten the first strike in, a slash with a knife that was designed to shock, disfigure, and terrify me. It worked.

What brought me some thirty miles from my home to fight in the parking lot of a pool hall? My buddy's name was on the line. He was losing face, so I decided that I needed to defend him. It was a matter of friendship, of honor. So, in my senior year of high school, five close friends and I cut the deal for a fight—five on five at the appointed pool hall—and just to add drama, we were going to do it at midnight.

I got there early to hang out with my buddies and so we could amp ourselves up for the confrontation. It was maybe a quarter to midnight when I stepped outside for a smoke. One of the three guys hanging around near the door gave me a hard look and then spat out, "Wadda you looking at?" "Nothing," I replied, and turned to go back inside. I heard one of them move and looked back to see what was going on when I was met by a knife slash across my face, striking my teeth and making my mouth an "X" instead of the nice, straight line my momma gave me. When I felt that blade grate across my teeth, I knew I was in trouble, and then my lower lip fell open like overcooked chicken dropping from the bone.

This wasn't the glorious battle I'd imagined. It was pain and blood and terror. What would the victor get from this fight? Absolutely nothing! No turf, no money, nothing, save perhaps a little pride. And the loser? I wound up with eighty stitches and a missing tooth. It cost me a day in the hospital, a big medical bill, and this scar you are looking at right now.

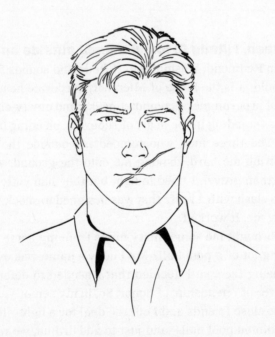

Introduction

> Spitting blood
> clears up reality
> and dream alike.
> —SUNAO (1887-1926)[1]

When someone uses the word *fight*, in your head you might picture something like a boxing match. A squaring off of two gentlemen with differences. There would be rules, and it would have a beginning and an end. But that's not what fighting is.

Violence is everywhere—on the street, in the workplace, on campus, and in the community. It can be instigated by everyone from drunken fools who hit like Jell-O to drug-crazed lunatics who can not only throw a good punch but will slash your throat for good measure.

You might be the instigator, the victim, a witness, any or all of the above. You might see violence coming or it might catch you totally by surprise. Aggression can come from friends, relatives, acquaintances, or total strangers. It can be logical or illogical, easily predictable or totally unexpected. It might be some crack-head trying to score a few bucks for his next rock, an irate driver in the grip of road rage, or a neighborhood bully intimidating you to make his point. Or it might be your drunken brother at your cousin's wedding, or it might be your best friend having a drug reaction at a party.

Aggression doesn't have to make sense at the time and often won't. Whenever the face of violence is glaring at you with that cold, hard stare, however, you must deal with it effectively in order to survive. For example, a friend of ours was putting some dishes away one afternoon when his sister tried to kill him with a steak knife. One moment he was leaning over the dishwasher and the next there was a wedge of razor-sharp steel whistling toward his lower back. Why? She simply wanted to know what it would be like to murder someone, though he did not know that, nor frankly care about that, at the time. All he was concerned with was not dying. Fortunately, he caught a reflection in his peripheral vision, reacted appropriately, disarmed her, and survived unscathed.

That's where situational awareness comes into play. If you see violence coming early enough, you can get out of its path. With sufficient warning to prepare yourself mentally and physically, you can choose to fight or not to fight. When you are caught by surprise, however, you frequently have no choice but to fight . . . and on his terms rather than yours. Predators don't want to fight, they want to *win*.

Escape and survival are admirable goals. Self-defense really isn't about fighting like most people think. Self-defense is about not being there when the other guy wants to fight. Fighting is a participatory event, which means you were part of the problem. Even if you think you were only "defending" yourself, if your actions contributed to the creation, escalation, and execution of violence, then you were fighting. And fighting is illegal and a really bad idea.

So what good can come of fighting? Perhaps you "win," beating the other guy down with your fists. But you'll often find that the guy you just beat will come back with a weapon, or with friends, or with a lawyer or the police. And that's the upside of winning. If you get the worst of a fight, the best you can hope for is a few bruises. But it's not unusual to suffer injuries that are far more serious. Go visit an emergency room in an urban area on a Friday or Saturday night and you'll see what we mean.

The brutal reality of a violent encounter is that if you wind up in a position where you can no longer defend yourself during a fight, you are at the other guy's mercy. Often, there is only a thin veneer of civilization, laws written on paper and enforced by folks who are much too far away to intervene right here, right now, standing between you and his wrath. He may choose to break off the fight when you are curled up into a little ball of agony at his feet. Or he may decide to put the boots to you.

Hollywood Fantasy vs. Brutal Reality

The realities of street violence are different from what most people think. The boxing match or mixed martial arts tournament pales in comparison to the brutality of a street fight. Sure, competitors do get seriously hurt from time to time in the ring, but these competitions are first and foremost sporting events. To help ensure the safety of everyone involved, competitors use various types of gear, such as padded gloves, mouth guards, and groin protection.

Unlike actual street fighting, sporting competitions have weight classes. Take the Ultimate Fighting Championship (UFC), for instance. Under its rules, competitors are grouped into divisions: lightweight (over 145 pounds to 155 pounds), welterweight (over 155 to 170 pounds), middleweight (over 170 to 185 pounds), light heavyweight (over 185 to 205 pounds), and heavyweight (over 205 to 265 pounds). On the street, you may find yourself tangling with someone much larger or smaller than yourself, or more than one adversary simultaneously.

Sporting competitions have set time periods. Sticking with

XXI

the UFC example, non-championship bouts run three rounds, while championship matches last five, each five minutes in duration. They have a one-minute rest period between rounds. On the street, fights rarely last more than a few seconds, but when they do, there is no stopping until it's done, someone intercedes, or the authorities arrive to break things up.

In the ring, you can win by submission (tap or verbal), knockout, technical knockout, decision, disqualification, or forfeiture. On the street, you win by surviving.

Unlike brawling on the street, so-called "no holds barred" events have a whole lot of rules. Take that literally: They bar no holds, yet they do ban lots of other stuff. Stuff that can be effective on the street, particularly if you are a smaller and/or weaker combatant. The UFC, for example, outlaws the following:

- Head butts
- Eye gouges
- Throat strikes
- Grabbing the trachea
- Biting
- Hair pulling
- Groin striking
- Fish hooking
- Putting your finger into any orifice or into any cut or laceration on an opponent
- Small joint manipulation
- Striking to the spine
- Striking the back of the head
- Striking downward with the point of your elbow
- Clawing, pinching, or twisting the opponent's flesh
- Grabbing the clavicle
- Kicking the head of a grounded opponent
- Kneeing the head of a grounded opponent
- Stomping a grounded opponent
- Kicking the other guy's kidney with your heel
- Spiking an opponent to the canvas so that he lands on his head or neck
- Throwing an opponent out of the ring
- Holding the shorts or gloves of an opponent
- Spitting at an opponent
- Engaging in an "unsportsmanlike" conduct that causes an injury to an opponent
- Holding the ropes or the fence
- Using abusive language in the ring or fenced area
- Attacking an opponent during a break period
- Attacking an opponent who is under the care of the referee
- Attacking an opponent after the bell has sounded the end of a period
- Disregarding the referee's instructions
- Interference by someone in the competitor's corner.

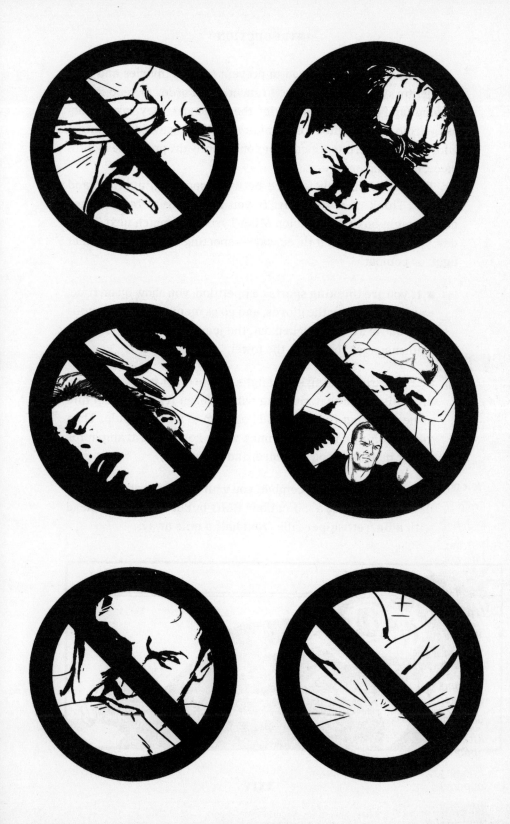

These rules are designed to prevent serious injuries and give competitors a sporting chance to succeed. In order to keep things moving (and more interesting for the audience), they take points away from a competitor for "timidity," including avoiding contact with an opponent, intentionally or consistently dropping the mouthpiece, or faking an injury.

There is a huge difference between sparring, fighting, and combat. Think of it this way. If you are going to face former heavyweight boxing champion Mike Tyson in a match next Tuesday, you can approach it three ways—sporting competition, street fight, or combat.

- If you are thinking sports competition, you show up on time, weigh in, strap on the gloves, and go as many as twelve rounds until one of you is knocked out, the judges make a decision, or your manager throws in the towel.

- If you are thinking street fight, on the other hand, you show up at his house that morning with a dozen friends, jump him as he walks out the door, and beat him to a bloody pulp. Then you kick him a few more times while he's down, trample his flower beds for good measure, and drive away.

- If you are thinking combat, you wait outside his house Monday night and put a .50-caliber BMG bullet through his head with a Barrett sniper rifle from half a mile away.

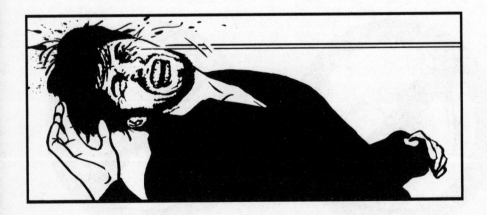

A bit of disparity between those scenarios, huh? Street fights are much more like combat than sports competition. Slickly choreographed Hollywood films only feed the fantasy of what true violence entails. Beware these misconceptions. Don't confuse sports with combat or misconstrue entertainment as reality.

Size and Intensity Are Not the Same Thing

There is a famous saying, originally attributed to author Mark Twain, that goes, "It is not the size of the dog in the fight, but the size of the fight in the dog." Often quoted, this maxim is absolutely true.

For example, in 1942 Audie Murphy (1924–71) tried to enlist in the military at the outset of World War II. He was turned down by both the United States Marines and the paratroopers for being too small—Murphy stood five feet five inches tall and was 110 pounds. When the army finally accepted him, they tried to make him serve as a cook . . . until he reached the battlefield.

In two years of service at the European front during World War II, Murphy killed 240 German soldiers in documented firefights. He won the Medal of Honor, the Distinguished Service Cross, the Legion of Merit, the Silver Star (twice), and the Bronze Star Medal (twice). He was also awarded the Purple Heart three times for combat injuries plus a variety of other honors totaling some thirty-two medals. This made him America's most decorated combat veteran.

How did a scrawny eighteen-year-old boy named Audie from Texas do it? Despite his small stature, he was one tough SOB. His father deserted the family when he was a small child. Only nine of his twelve brothers and sisters lived past the age of eighteen. His mother died when he was sixteen, leaving him in charge, and he gave up the three remaining kids to an orphanage.

He had a rough life that might have broken a lesser man, yet it forged a mental toughness that far outweighed his physical build. He was resilient too, tough enough to jump up on a burning

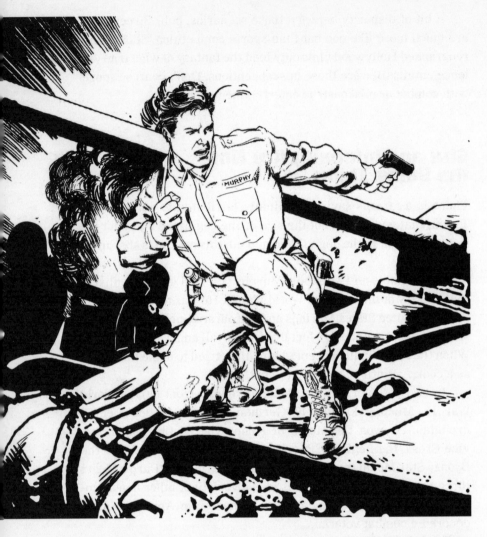

tank and use a .50-caliber machine gun to hold off advancing German troops, killing fifty, all while he bled from a leg wound.

Next time you equate size with intensity, remember the guy you are about to square off with might have had a rougher life than Audie Murphy. If so, you are about to find out what *intensity* really means.

Since the best way to win a fight is not to get in one, the first section of this book is all about becoming aware of and learning how to avoid violent confrontations. It explains some of the brutal realities of violence so that you'll think twice about fighting too.

Unfortunately, there are instances when you have no choice but to fight and others where it is prudent to do so. In those situations, you need to know how to do it effectively. The second section of this book is about what actually happens during a violent encounter, helping you understand smart things you might want to try and dumb things you should avoid during a fight.

The last section covers the aftermath of violence, showing that it's almost never over when it's over. Surviving the fight is just the beginning. There is a host of other consequences to address, including first aid, managing witnesses, finding a good attorney, interacting with law enforcement, and dealing with psychological trauma.

A key aspect of this book is the checklist in the next section, entitled "How Far Am I Willing to Go?" To use this checklist properly *stop reading this book now and fill in your answers. Once you have finished reading the book, go back and do it again.* There is no answer key. There is no right or wrong when it comes to responding to these questions. This exercise is designed to make you think, putting the information you are about to read into a context that will be meaningful for you when you must make decisions under threat in the real world. Once you have finished reading the book, see what you have learned, evaluate if and how your attitude has changed, and reflect on what you might do next time you run across aggressive or violent behavior on the street.

Our goal is to help you put things into perspective and give you the tools necessary to navigate the world of violence without running into any insurmountable challenges along your way. It's a serious topic, yet we have tried to make it interesting, meaningful, and, most of all, thought provoking. After all, knowledge and good sense are your main weapons of self-defense.

How Far Am I Willing to Go?

You need to think about what you're willing to do, what you are not willing to do, and what you are willing to have done to you. Such decisions cannot be made during a tense, dangerous encounter. Below is a list of scenarios.

There is always a cost in physical and/or emotional well-being to taking action as well as not taking action. There is no right or wrong answer. The important thing is to evaluate realistically where you stand.

At minimum, this questionnaire should be completed before *and* after you read this book. Use a pencil or make a photocopy so that you can do it twice. It is a good idea to reevaluate periodically too.

Check the appropriate boxes in each column.

- ☐ Admit when I am wrong and sincerely apologize
- ☐ Allow myself to be blindfolded
- ☐ Allow myself to be captured by a criminal and moved to a secondary crime scene
- ☐ Allow myself to be tied up to live a little longer
- ☐ Allow others to call me names without responding
- ☐ Avoid a place (for example, neighborhood, pool hall, nightclub, public park, eatery) where a specific race or ethnic group congregates
- ☐ Avoid a place (for example, street corner, housing complex, store, area in a mall, fast-food restaurant, tavern) where there might be trouble
- ☐ Ban someone from my home and/or place of business
- ☐ Be raped
- ☐ Be stolen from
- ☐ Be threatened by a loved one
- ☐ Be threatened by a stranger

- ☐ Call 911 (or local emergency number) to report a crime in progress
- ☐ Carry a knife or a firearm on a daily basis
- ☐ Chase a thief or other criminal in my car
- ☐ Chase a thief or other criminal on foot
- ☐ Cooperate with the police
- ☐ Defend a weaker friend
- ☐ Defend a weaker stranger
- ☐ Defend my honor
- ☐ Eliminate contact with a friend, relative, or acquaintance who is a known troublemaker
- ☐ Fight a group by myself
- ☐ Fight one-on-one
- ☐ Fight over an insult to my favorite sports team
- ☐ Fight when I drink or use drugs
- ☐ Gouge out someone's eye in self-defense
- ☐ Hand over my hard-earned money to a mugger

- [ ] Interfere in another person's argument
- [ ] Join a gang
- [ ] Just walk away from a potential problem no matter how much others might criticize me for it
- [ ] Kick someone when he's down
- [ ] Kill in self-defense
- [ ] Kill a close friend or relative in self-defense
- [ ] Let my car be broken into or defaced
- [ ] Let my personal items be broken or defaced
- [ ] Listen attentively, even when I am angry
- [ ] Lose face in private, in front of a close friend, relative, or significant other
- [ ] Lose face in public amongst friends or acquaintances
- [ ] Lose face in public amongst strangers
- [ ] Maim, permanently disable, or kill another person in self-defense
- [ ] Own a weapon
- [ ] Participate in a mob
- [ ] Physically intervene in a fight
- [ ] Report another student or coworker who is carrying a weapon on the premises
- [ ] Report another student or coworker who is making threats to harm others
- [ ] See another person's position
- [ ] Sell drugs
- [ ] Shoot a person in self-defense, knowing that he might die or be crippled for life
- [ ] Show respect
- [ ] Stab a person in self-defense, knowing that he might die or be crippled for life
- [ ] Strike first if I feel that violence is imminent
- [ ] Take risks such as cutting off other drivers, tailgating, or traveling through undesirable neighborhoods in order to save time on my commute
- [ ] Testify in court against a violent offender whose crimes I have witnessed, even if he threatens retribution
- [ ] Threaten another person to get what I want
- [ ] Train in a martial art like karate, tae kwon do, or boxing
- [ ] Turn my back to an armed individual when ordered to do so
- [ ] Use a weapon to injure or kill another person
- [ ] Use anything as a weapon to protect my life or another's life
- [ ] Use whatever force is necessary to neutralize an adult who is threatening me with a weapon
- [ ] Use whatever force is necessary to neutralize a child who is threatening me with a weapon
- [ ] Visit a location (for example, street corner, housing complex, store, nightclub, restaurant, or tavern) where violence has recently occurred
- [ ] Visit a location (for example, street corner, housing complex, store, nightclub, restaurant, or tavern) where violence is common or has recently occurred
- [ ] Watch a loved one be beaten down without intervening
- [ ] Watch a loved one be kidnapped or taken hostage without intervening
- [ ] Watch a loved one be murdered without physically intervening
- [ ] Watch a loved one be raped without intervening
- [ ] Watch a stranger be beaten down without intervening
- [ ] Watch a stranger be kidnapped or taken hostage without intervening
- [ ] Watch a stranger be murdered without intervening
- [ ] Watch a stranger be raped without intervening

HOW TO WIN A FIGHT

BEFORE VIOLENCE OCCURS

> When autumn winds blow
> not one leaf remains
> the way it was.
> —TOGYU (1705-1749)[2]

Rule number one of self-defense is "Don't get hit." Sounds simple, right? But if you're in a fight, you're going to get hit. So the only way to not get hit is to not be there when there's a fight. That means avoiding situations or locations where violence is most likely to occur. Is it easy to stay out of crime-ridden housing projects? Probably. But how many times have you been drinking alcohol at a sporting event, surrounded by thousands of other drunken fans? A fight is more likely to break out there than in the projects.

Let's face it: We do risky things from time to time. We walk home alone through unfamiliar neighborhoods. We yell at other drivers on the road. Most times nothing bad happens, so we never get feedback that, yes, eventually something will happen.

Most people who find themselves involved in violence think that they were just minding their own business and suddenly this problem came out of nowhere. It just seems like this at the time, though. There is always some type of buildup, something they didn't see or didn't recognize the significance of until it was too late. That's why it appears to have come out of nowhere. Oftentimes what you think is an innocent comment, gesture, or look is what gets you clobbered.

Self-defense is about keeping your cool, not being the instigator, even inadvertently. It's about paying attention, being aware of and evading threats before it's too late. Less ideally, if the violence is right in front of you, it's about doing all you can to avoid a fight. The only fight you know you'll win, the one you are guaranteed to walk away from with all your parts and pieces fully intact, is the fight you never get into. This is what Sun Tzu meant when he wrote, "To subdue an enemy without fighting is the highest skill."

CHAPTER ONE

Awareness Is Your Best Defense

The best self-defense is being aware of and avoiding dangerous people and hazardous situations. The cornerstone of self-defense is having a solid understanding of time and place and how they relate to you and others around you. In some ways, it's more an attitude than a skill. Any time you are near others, it pays to be vigilant, striking a balance between obliviousness and paranoia. If you can sense danger before stumbling across it, you have a better chance of escaping unscathed.

Think about it this way: Nine out of ten dangers can be identified and avoided simply by learning how to look out for them. Since it is still possible to talk your way out of more than half of the potentially violent situations that you do get yourself into, this means that you should only need to fight your way out of three, four, or at worst, five of every hundred hazardous encounters. With good situational awareness, you may never have anywhere near a hundred such confrontations in your lifetime. Those odds aren't all that bad, huh?

Knowing when it is time to leave a party is an example of good situational awareness. Fights tend to happen after a certain time of night. It's not the hour on the clock that's important, but rather the mood of the crowd. Most people have a good time and leave long before the shit starts. Just about everyone who's going to hook up has already done so and is off having fun. As the crowd starts to thin, those who have nothing better to do than cause trouble are the ones who are left. Buzzing with frustration and raging hormones, those who insist on hanging on well into the night are the ones who get caught up in violence.

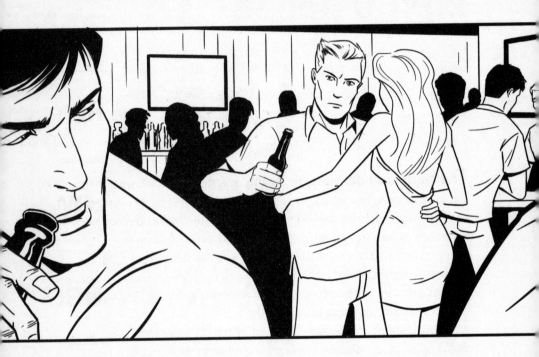

The same thing applies on the street. Criminals may be scary, but they are neither exceptionally bright nor hardworking. We are stereotyping here, but seriously, how many rocket scientists or Mensa members are there on death row? Many crimes are quick-fix substitutes for earning a living the old-fashioned way. Why, then, would a street thug go out of his way to tangle with a tough, prepared target when easier prey is readily available?

By surveying and evaluating your environment, you achieve control over what happens to you. Good situational awareness helps you make yourself a hard target by eliminating easy opportunities for those who wish to do you harm. It's not a guarantee of perfect safety, since there truly are no absolutes when it comes to self-defense, yet situational awareness will keep you safer.

It's as simple as paying attention to your built-in survival mechanisms. And it can be refined and improved through practice. Can you remember a time when you were driving along the highway, suddenly "knew" the car beside you was going to swerve into your lane, and took evasive action to avoid an accident? It is so common that most people forget about such incidents shortly after they happen, but this ability to predict what other drivers are going to do is an example of learning good situational awareness.

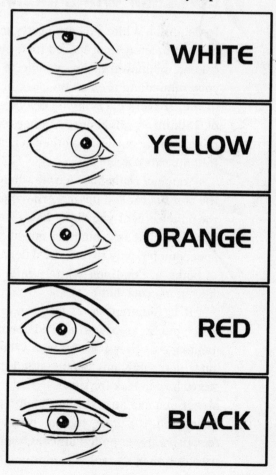

Constant vigilance is emotionally and physically draining. No one can maintain an elevated level of awareness at all times in all places. There is a difference between being aware and becoming paranoid. Consequently, many self-defense experts use a color code system to help define and communicate appropriate levels of situational awareness for whatever situation people could find themselves in.

The most commonly used approach, codified by Colonel Jeff Cooper, was based in large part on the color alert system developed by the United States Marine Corps during World War II and later modified for civilian use. These color code conditions include White (oblivious), Yellow (aware), Orange (alert), Red (concerned), and Black (under attack).

The mind-set and attitude of each condition are described below. Think of each condition as a distinct state along a continuum, but don't get too hung up on each level. The important concept is that the tactical situations you face will warrant various amounts of vigilance.

Condition White (Oblivious)

In Condition White, you are pretty much ignoring your surroundings, completely unprepared for trouble if it arrives. You are distracted or unaware, thus unable to perceive existing danger in your immediate area or be alert for any that may be presented to you. Drivers carrying on conversations with passengers, people talking on cell phones, runners wearing headphones and jamming to their music, and other generally preoccupied individuals fall into this category.

You may remember a time when you were driving along with the stereo cranked up and grooving to the music when suddenly the police officer you didn't know was behind you set off his siren and lights. Nearly jumping out of your skin, you checked your speedometer, only to find you'd been speeding. That's an example of being in Condition White. While almost everyone has done it, it's not too cool, huh?

It is illuminating to watch a crowd at a mall, nightclub, or other public area with a predator mind-set. Read people's body language as they pass by you. Who looks like a victim and who does not? Oblivious people stand out from the crowd once you know how to look for them.

If you are attacked in Condition White, you are likely going to be hurt. If armed, you can easily become a danger to yourself or others. Even police officers, who have access to much better training than the average civilian, have been killed by their own weapons when they relaxed their vigilance at the wrong times or places.*

Condition Yellow (Aware)

Although you are not looking for or even expecting trouble in Condition Yellow, if it comes up, you will have a good chance to identify it in time to react. You can identify, without looking twice, generally who and what is around you—vehicles, people, building entrances, street corners, and areas that might provide concealment and/or cover† should something untoward happen.

Body language is important. You should be self-assured and appear confident in everything you do, yet not present an overt challenge or threat to others. You walk with your head up, casually scanning your immediate area as well as what is just beyond. Someone in Condition Yellow sees who and what is ahead of them, is aware of their environment to each side, and occasionally turns to scan behind them. If you make eye contact and then lift your gaze, it may come across as haughty, whereas lowering your gaze may appear meek, so your eyes should move side to side as you scan. Avoid potentially confrontational stares and weak, furtive glances by continuously taking in the scene around you without stopping on any one thing unless it appears threatening.

Condition Yellow is appropriate any time you're in public. If you are armed, it is essential. You should notice anything out of place, anyone looking or acting in an unusual manner, or anything that is out of context, to evaluate for potential threat. Examples might include a crowd gathered for no apparent reason, someone wearing heavy clothing on a summer day, a person studiously

---

* For example, on November 29, 2009, felon Maurice Clemmons murdered four Lakewood, Washington, police officers—Sergeant Mark Renninger and officers Ronald Owens, Tina Griswold, and Greg Richards—at a Forza coffee shop.

† Something that offers concealment (e.g., a bush) keeps bad guys from seeing you but does not provide physical protection, while cover (e.g., a stone wall) can keep both the bad guy and/or his weapon from getting to you.

avoiding eye contact, anyone whose hands are hidden from view, a person moving awkwardly or with an unusual gait, or someone who simply stares at you for no apparent reason. Anything that stimulates your intuitive survival sense should be studied more closely.

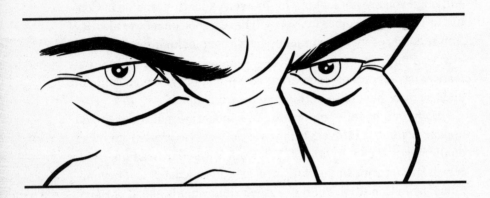

Condition Orange (Alert)

People in Condition Orange have become aware of some nonspecific danger and need to ascertain whether there is a legitimate threat to their safety. You may have heard a shout, the sound of glass breaking, or an unidentified sudden noise where you would not have expected one. You might also have seen another person or a group of people acting abnormally, someone whose demeanor makes you feel uncomfortable, or somebody whose appearance or behavior stands out as unusual.

In this state, you should focus on the possible danger, but not to the exclusion of a broader awareness of your surroundings. Trouble may be starting in other places in addition to the one that has drawn your attention (e.g., an ambush). It may be prudent to reposition yourself to take advantage of cover and escape routes should it become necessary to use them. If unarmed, you should also try to spot objects that can be used as makeshift weapons or distractions, but it is premature to make any aggressive moves at this point.

If armed, it is a good idea to be sure that your weapon is accessible, though it is not prudent to call attention to it yet. If in a lonely area like a parking garage, bathroom, or alley, it is usually wise to move into a better-lit or more populated area. Denying the privacy for criminal acts to occur or escalate is one of the fundamentals of self-defense.

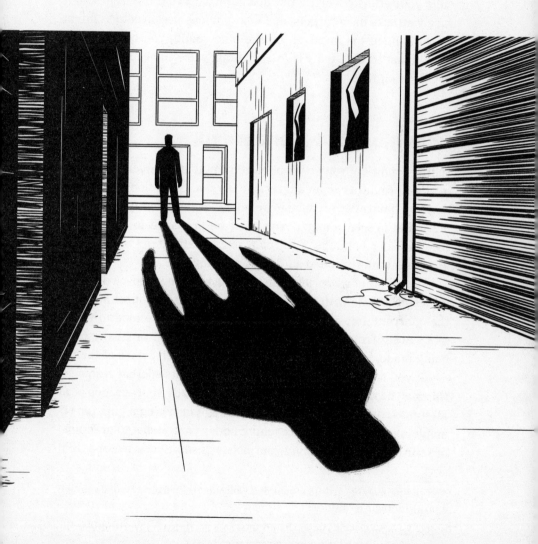

This is also a good time to prepare a plan of action, contemplating what you might have to do should the danger become an imminent threat. If the trouble is immediate but not directed at you, it may be prudent to move to safety* and then call for help.

If, on the other hand, it turns out that trouble is not brewing, you simply return to Condition Yellow, abandoning the plan. Consider your effort good practice and go on with your day. A predator rarely attacks hard targets, and your obvious preparedness might have changed his mind. If, on the other hand, you become convinced that trouble truly is forthcoming, you will need to escalate to Condition Red.

Condition Red (Concerned)

In this condition, you've encountered a potential adversary or are in close proximity to an aggressive person. Condition Red means that you have every reason to believe that the other guy(s) pose a clear and present danger. You must be prepared to fight, hopefully taking advantage of the plan you visualized in Condition Orange (assuming you had sufficient warning).

At this point it is prudent to begin moving away toward escape routes, locations with strategic cover, or areas of concealment. If the confrontation is immediate, it is often a good idea to try to move away from any weapons being brandished or distractions being made, while at the same time keeping well aware of them.

If you are armed and the situation warrants a lethal response, this may be the point where you draw and ready your weapon or at least make its presence known.† If you are carrying a gun, for example, this might include reaching under your jacket to grab hold of your pistol and thumbing your holster's safety release. A verbal

---

* If the combatants overhear your call, you may inadvertently make yourself a target of their wrath.

† See chapter 6, "Use Only as Much Force as the Situation Warrants," to understand when lethal force may be appropriate.

challenge at this point, such as telling the adversary to back off, may prove useful if time permits. De-escalation may still be an option but it can also backfire, so you must be prepared in case it does not work. While a show of ability and readiness to resist with countervailing force may stop the confrontation, it could also elevate it to the next level.

Condition Black (Under Attack)

This is a fight. Although it is possible to skip instantly from Condition Yellow up to Condition Black, encounters generally escalate at a pace at which you can adjust your level of awareness incrementally so long as you did not start off in Condition White. This gives observant individuals a leg up in dealing with dangerous adversaries.

Once you have been assaulted, verbal challenges and de-escalation attempts are no longer useful. You must flee or fight back. If armed and confronted by an armed attacker or multiple unarmed assailants, you may decide to use your weapon in self-defense. Shooting to "wound" and firing "warning" shots are Hollywood folderol; any time you pull the trigger, it's serious business. The same thing goes for knives, blunt instruments, and other impromptu weapons as well.

Be sure that you are legally, ethically, and morally entitled to do so before employing countervailing force. Your intent must be to stop the assault that is in progress so that you can escape to safety or otherwise remain safe until help arrives. You must not want to kill or hurt anyone nor teach him a lesson. Such attitudes can make you the aggressor in the eyes of the law. In addition, even if you are never charged with a crime, you will still have to live with yourself afterward.

Each encounter will be different, so your tactics will change accordingly. It is vital to use sufficient force to control the situation and keep yourself safe without overreacting. You will, no doubt, want to treat a drunken relative at a family reunion quite differently than a homicidal street punk coming at you in a drug-induced rage. We'll talk more about this in section 2.

Know When He's Eager to Hit You

Violence rarely happens in a vacuum. There is always some escalation process—even a really short one—that precedes it. Before the fight is the "interview." This is where the other guy sizes you up and determines whether or not you will be an easy mark. If you seem like a mark when he glares at you, he might move to verbal insults. If he still feels confident, he could move to shoving. No two encounters are the same, but there are clear signs of escalation before the majority of violent encounters.

Insults and other forms of verbal abuse are common precursors to a fight. Oftentimes, the other guy is trying to intimidate you. He might also be trying to goad you into throwing the first blow so that he has a legitimate excuse to stomp a mud hole in you. Swallow your pride and walk away if you can. The more dangerous you are, the less you should feel a need to prove it.

There are two types of aggressors who might confront you on the street: dominance attackers and predators. Dominance attackers want to feel superior to their victim. If you walk away from one of these individuals, he will usually let you go in peace. He feels that he has won by making you back down. Predatory attackers, on the other hand, want a victim who will not put up a fight. If you walk away from one of these individuals, you may trigger the very attack you were trying to avoid.

But trying to leave puts you on better legal ground if you ultimately have to fight back, particularly if witnesses observe what happened or the incident ends up being captured on film or video. With the prevalence of closed-circuit security monitors, cell phone cameras, traffic cams, and other forms of electronic surveillance out there, that's a common situation.

While the escalation process varies from encounter to encounter, there are certain common behaviors that may lead to violence. Possible trouble indicators include:

- *Glaring, staring, or otherwise "sizing you up"*
- *Attempts by an individual or group to follow, herd (control your direction), flank, or mirror your movements*
- *Making unprovoked accusations, threats, aggressive requests or demands, or using foul language for no apparent reason*
- *Baiting or attempting to provoke an aggressive response from you (for example, "What's your problem?" or "What are you looking at?")*
- *Moving into a range that enables the other guy to attack, particularly when the movements are covert or sudden*
- *Unusual or out-of-place body movements, aggressive gestures, agitated pacing, clenched fists, forward weight shift, straightening the spine, or adopting a fighting stance*
- *Clearing space to move or draw a weapon*
- *Hands and/or teeth clenched, a taut neck, or other stiff or shaking body movements*
- *Shouting to startle or paralyze you as an attack begins*

While it is common to experience this type of obvious escalation, ambushes also occur. In such situations, the escalation has already occurred, yet the victim is unaware of it because it took place solely within the mind of the attacker. He has already looked you over, conducted a mental interview to ascertain that you are an easy target, and decided upon a course of action against you. This summing up can cause a situation where you have no choice but to fight.

Regrettably, most people are not mentally prepared to react to sudden violence, so are needlessly hurt or killed despite the fact that they saw it coming. It does not matter why you were attacked, simply that you *were* attacked. Do not deny what is happening at the time, but rather respond appropriately to defend yourself. Worry about making sense of the encounter afterward.

As a general rule, you should err on the side of caution, trying to avoid or evade problem situations before they spin out of control. It is important to trust your instincts in such situations. Whether you see it or not, there will often be some indicator that can warn you of a person's intent just before they attack.

This indicator is often called the "tell." Poker players coined this term, which refers to some movement or gesture that lets them figure out when an opponent is bluffing. In the self-defense community, the tell has been called many things, such as the "adrenal dump" or the "twitch." If you do not see the tell, you are bound to lose. Even if you are really, really quick, action is always faster than reaction. Missing the tell is what gets you sucker punched.

The tell involves small physical movements a person might

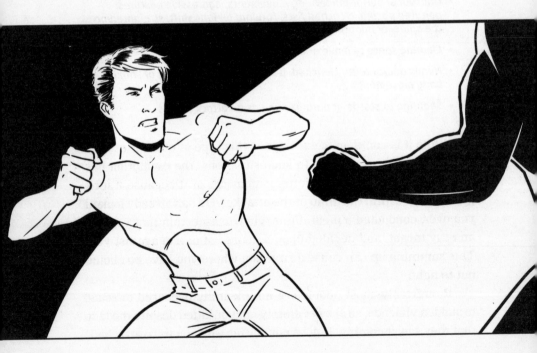

make to signal intent to attack as well as subtle changes in the person's energy. These indicators could include a slight drop of the shoulder, a tensing of the neck, or a puckering of the lips. That's tough to spot, though changes in the person's energy can be more readily identified:

- *A person who was standing still moves slightly. A weight shift is far subtler than a step, but the change could signal preparation for attack.*

- *A sudden pallor or sudden flushing of the person's face (that is, an adrenaline-induced vasoconstriction).*

- *A person who was looking at you suddenly looks away or, conversely, a person who was looking away suddenly makes eye contact.*

- *A change in the rate, tone, pitch, or volume of a person's voice, such as when someone who is shouting becomes suddenly quiet or, conversely, one who has been quiet begins raising his or her voice.*

- *A sudden change in the person's breathing (i.e., shallow and fast for untrained adversaries, slow and deep for trained opponents).*

By understanding the indicators of a potential attack, you will have a better opportunity to avoid confrontations and defend yourself effectively. Action being faster than reaction, the earlier you identify these indicators, the better prepared and safer you will be.

Don't Get Caught Up in the Escalato Follies

Escalato follies refers to the one-upmanship cycle that almost inevitably leads to violence unless one party backs down and breaks off the game. The term *escalato* was originally coined by musician, comedian, and political satirist Tom Lehrer to describe the process of irrational commitment in which people continue to increase their investment in a decision despite knowing that it was the wrong thing to do. The current term in business and political circles is *escalation of commitment*. It is also very closely tied to threat displays, which are things you do hoping the other guy will back off, so you won't need to use violence. Sometimes they work, sometimes they make it worse.

You know the drill—you think I just ogled your girlfriend's ass, so you glare at me. I was actually minding my own business, nursing a beer and spacing out, so I don't know what the heck you're pissed off about and flip you the bird in response. Now you're really mad because I'm a serious dickhead, so you get in my face and start spewing insults. I'm not about to let you get away with that, so I toss my beer in your face. You haul back to hit me but I beat you to the draw and kick you in the 'nads. You stumble backward, grab a pool cue, and bust it over my head.

Things go downhill from there. By the time the dust settles, one of us is carried out on a gurney while the other gets to wear a

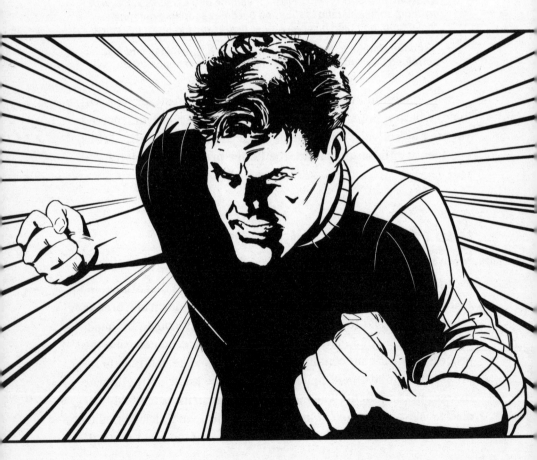

stainless steel bracelet, earns a trip to the local police department, takes out a second mortgage to cover legal expenses, and quickly discovers that he's seriously screwed up his life.

While this example might seem silly, this kind of scenario plays itself out all the time in real life. These escalato follies are a supremely dangerous game—one you really, really do not want to play. Win or lose, there's always a cost to it.

One way to avoid getting caught up in this is by knowing how to respond rather than react. Responding is a planned course of action, one that leaves you in control of your emotions and actions. Reacting, on the other hand, cedes control to the opponent. If you become angry, defensive, or emotionally involved, it is easy to get caught up in the cycle.

Even if the other guy is a complete ass, losing face while remaining alive and free is far better than fighting to prove you're right. He's acting like an ass because he wants you to react to it. If you do, you've let him dictate your actions.

Do you want to be responsible for an accidental death because you lost your temper? Even if you are not charged with a crime, could you live with yourself afterward, knowing that you've taken a life and destroyed a family? While it may be pretty easy to rationalize what you did, justifying your actions in your own mind for the first few years, it's really tough to wake up to the knowledge that you are a killer every day for the rest of your life.

Avoid the escalato follies at all costs. Keep your ego in check. In addition, do your best to verbally de-escalate a confrontation, talking your way out of trouble before the confrontation becomes violent. Apologizing for some perceived slight, even when you did nothing wrong, often beats the alternative.

You may be saying to yourself, "Come on, man, dying from a fist-fight? That's outrageous." It is not only possible, it happens all the time.

For example, Mark Leidheisl, thirty-nine, a regional senior vice president for Wells Fargo Bank, died on April 20, 2005, from a blunt force trauma injury to the head. Sacramento police reported that the incident that led to Leidheisl's death might have been fueled by road rage and that he appeared to have been the aggressor. An unmarked medicine bottle in Leidheisl's car contained Paxil (an antidepressant), morphine (a powerful painkiller), and an unidentified third pill type. Tests later found that he had a blood alcohol level of at least 0.13 (more than the legal driving limit of 0.08) and opiates in his system. Drugs, alcohol, and violence frequently go together, with very bad results.

Here's what happened: Reports state that Leidheisl cut off another vehicle while driving out of Arco Arena's parking lot after attending a Sacramento Kings game. Leidheisl and his friend exchanged heated words with the two men in the other vehicle. Then both cars stopped on a nearby street, and all four men got out of their vehicles. During the subsequent fight, Leidheisl fell and hit his head on the pavement, causing the fatal injury. The suspects from the other vehicle, ages forty-three and forty-four, left the scene but contacted police after seeing news reports about how seriously Leidheisl was hurt.

District Attorney Jan Scully told reporters, "After a thorough review of the police investigation, it is clear that Mark Leidheisl died as a result of mutual combat between him and Jeffrey Berndt. One punch thrown in self-defense by Jeffrey Berndt struck Mark Leidheisl in the face, causing him to fall backward, striking his head on the asphalt pavement. This fall fractured Leidheisl's skull, causing his death."

A few moments of road rage and a guy was dead. Someone with a great career, a ton of friends, a wonderful family, and a whole lot to live for.

CHAPTER TWO

Don't Let Them Get into Position for Attack

Bad guys aren't going to pick a fight with someone when they stand a good chance of getting hurt in the process. Your adversary, therefore, will want to surprise and overwhelm you whenever possible. He may deploy a weapon as well. Furthermore, thugs sometimes work together in small groups to stack the odds even higher in their favor.

The good news is that the bad guys cannot hurt you if they cannot reach you. In order to pull off a successful attack, the other guy needs to close distance and move into a position from which he can strike. Fists, feet, knives, blunt instruments, and other hand-held weapons require close range to be effective. Even gunfights typically take place at close range. According to FBI statistics, about half of all gun murder victims are killed from a range of five feet or less.

Unless a lot of alcohol or drugs is involved, however, you will rarely be attacked in the middle of a crowd. Fringe areas adjacent to heavily traveled public places are where the majority of violent crimes occur. This includes areas such as parking lots, bathrooms, stairwells, laundry rooms, phone booths, ATM kiosks, and the like. Your level of awareness should be kicked up a notch whenever you travel through these fringe areas.

Pay attention to other individuals and behaviors that may constitute a threat. There are a variety of tactics that bad guys might use to get themselves into position to attack you. These include closing, cornering, surprising, pincering, herding, and surrounding.

Closing

The most common method of getting close enough to attack is simply walking up to the victim. This is often combined with some type of distraction, typically verbal, to help the bad guy seem less threatening while he maneuvers himself into position to strike.

There is no legitimate reason for a person you do not know to get closer than five feet from you on the street unless you are in the middle of a large crowd or sitting on public transportation. Trust your intuition. If he makes you uncomfortable and tries to close distance, warn him away. Don't worry about being rude or breaking some social norm. It is better to be a little embarrassed and safe than beaten to a pulp and sorry. After all, this is someone you've never met before and will likely never meet again.

Anyone who insists on closing after you have warned him away has clearly announced that his intentions are less than honorable. Demand space and be prepared to fight if it is not given.

Cornering

Cornering is a bit more strategic than simple closing. The bad guy angles his approach in a manner that traps you between him and a solid object such as the wall of a building or a parked vehicle. Indoors, he might block the only doorway into a room so that you need to go through him in order to escape.

A common cornering method is to approach a person when

he's getting into his car, particularly in mall parking lots, where he is carrying encumbering purchases and valuables such as cash and credit cards. Think about how long it takes to pull your keys out of your pocket, insert them into the lock, turn the lock, open the door, slip inside, close and lock the door, start up the vehicle, and drive away. You are vulnerable during most of those steps, trapped between the bad guy and your vehicle or stuck in the vehicle with the door open before you can get it closed and drive away.

Cornering behavior should always be a concern, particularly in fringe areas where attacks are more likely to occur. When traveling in these areas, pay close attention to alternate routes you might take in order to effect an escape. If your awareness is sufficient, you should be able to spot this behavior and move in an alternate direction before you can become trapped.

Surprising

Surprising requires a source of concealment from which the bad guy might spring when he chooses to attack. This can include trees, bushes, doorways, parked vehicles, garbage bins, or any other barriers behind which he can hide yet track your movements and step out to attack. Even pools of darkness between streetlights can be used for surprise if you are inattentive and the other guy is dressed appropriately.

Pay attention to your environment, particularly in areas you frequent, such as the sidewalk near your home, office, school, and so on. Look at these areas through the lens of a mugger. What are the sources of cover or concealment? If you were the bad guy, where would you hide? Once you know these locations, you can give them a quick once-over before you pass by, thwarting most surprise attacks.

Don't forget that he needs free access to be able to move out and attack you quickly, so he won't be in something like a garbage bin but rather hiding alongside it. Doors, on the other hand, facilitate rapid egress, so he could be sitting in a vehicle or standing behind the entrance to a building.

Pincering

Bad guys sometimes work together. The most common tactic is a pincer movement, in which one guy distracts you so that the other can sneak up on you from behind. The bad guys might split up as they approach you or spread out so that you pass one before being accosted by the other. That way one is already behind you when it goes down.

Be wary of individuals who "ping your radar" as you approach. Don't worry about embarrassing yourself by overreacting; just turn around and walk away. Similarly, if one or more individuals who were together split up as they approach you, angle off in another direction. If they start to follow, their intent will be clear. More often than not, your awareness marks you as a difficult target and they will find someone else to pick on.

Herding

Beyond the pincer movement, two or more thugs may employ a herding tactic. This is similar to what carnivores do in the wild. An individual makes his presence known in a manner that causes you enough concern for you to want to move to a safer location. As you attempt to flee, the bad guys control available routes along which you can travel in order to herd you toward a choke point where one or more members are waiting and planning to act. If you fail to take the hint and move, the assault takes place where you first made contact with the individual or group.

If you think you have thwarted this type of trap, it's a good idea to dial 911 or your local emergency number to report the suspicious activities. Just because you were able to avoid the ambush doesn't mean that the next guy who happens along will too.

As a good citizen, you can help others avoid becoming victims by drawing police attention to the area.

Surrounding

It gets even tougher when three or more bad guys work in concert. One will often try to distract you while the others move to surround you and cut off all avenues of escape. Typically, they will casually drift apart as you approach. Like the pincer movement, the group might also spread out so that you pass alongside them before being accosted. When you reach the midpoint of the group, the wings fold in to trap you.

Be wary of individuals who trigger your innate danger sense. If it is a large group, turn around and walk away. Listen for signs of pursuit and calmly check back over your shoulder after fifteen feet or so to see if they are starting to follow you. Do your best to show no fear but rather resolute preparedness. Fighting a large group is a losing proposition. Your best defense is to never get close enough to the bad guys to be in danger.

In all of these situations, the bad guy must close distance or control your movement in order to get into range to attack you. Don't let him do it.

CHAPTER THREE

Your Words Are a Weapon, Use Them Wisely

What you say during a tense encounter can determine whether you can walk away or whether you have to fight your way out of it. On the one hand, you might be able to verbally de-escalate a tense situation, while on the other, you can just as easily set the other guy off if you are not careful. Consequently, while

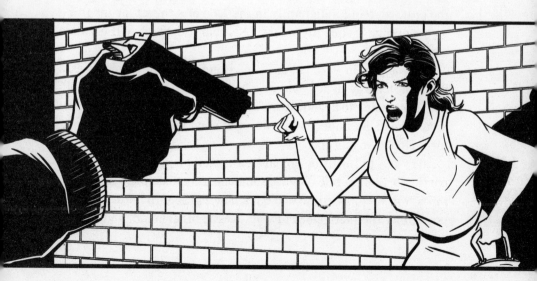

sticks and stones may break your bones, your words can actually kill you.

On January 27, 2005, actress Nicole duFresne was robbed at gunpoint on Manhattan's Lower East Side by nineteen-year-old Rudy Fleming, who stole her friend's purse and pistol-whipped her fiancé. What was supposed to be a simple property crime turned deadly, however, when the twenty-eight-year-old actress confronted the teenage robber. She became furious, shoved Fleming, and snapped, "What are you going to do, shoot us?" A fatal mistake—she was shot at point-blank range and died shortly thereafter in her fiancé's arms.

This tragedy is an excellent case study in what not to do when confronted by an armed aggressor. Experts often state that robbery is more often about power than anything else. Discussing the duFresne shooting, Alfonso Lenhardt of the National Crime Prevention Council said, "It's a tragedy, but in this case it sounds like the suspect felt he wasn't getting the respect he was due. When a gun is in the hands of a desperate person with low self-esteem, they're going to react that way."

Respect is paramount for gang members, even wannabes. Mouthing off to any street punk is dangerous. If you are confronted by an adversary, save your righteous indignation for a safer environment after the danger has passed. It does you no good to be right yet dead like duFresne. Having to be right despite the cost, reacting indignantly in the face of a threat, or insulting an adversary frequently guarantees that a conflict will escalate out of control.

If you are in error about something, admit it. Honesty is a much better way to de-escalate a bad situation than lying or stubbornly refusing to acknowledge a wrong. It is tough on the ego, but it sure beats an unnecessary hospital stay, jail time, or a premature trip to the morgue.

Try not to insult or embarrass the other person in any way, particularly in public. Giving someone a face-saving way out affords him the opportunity to back down gracefully. Put his back up against the metaphorical wall, on the other hand, and he will

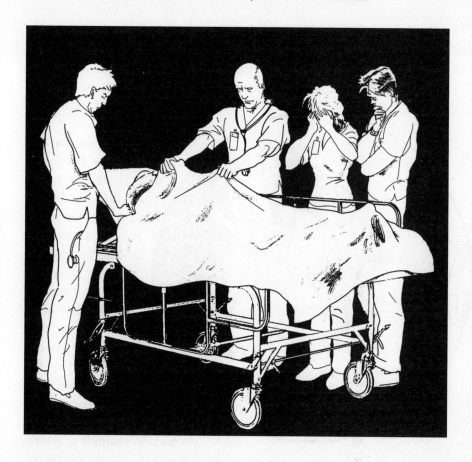

feel forced to lash out at you, striking back (from his perspective) to save his dignity and honor.

Even if you are in the right, it is sometimes prudent to pretend otherwise. Do not let your ego overrule your common sense. Giving your vehicle to a carjacker, your wallet to a robber, or your apology to someone who tries to start a fight hurts a lot less than eating a blade or a bullet.

Even if you cannot de-escalate a situation simply by talking, clever words may enable you to stall until help arrives or the attacker changes his mind and leaves. You can also use conversation as a psychological weapon to increase your chances of surviving or to create openings for your physical defenses. Deception, for example, is but one of the tactics you might choose to employ. Any convincing distraction you can create will be to your advantage, such as shouting for nonexistent friends. There is strength in numbers and in making an aggressor believe you are not alone.

If you realize that de-escalation is not working, it may also be possible to cause your opponent to make a mental twitch, providing a moment of opportunity to counterattack while he is mentally shifting gears. This twitch is brought about by dissonance between what the person expects and what you actually say or do.

A common example is asking a question. While the bad guy is focusing on your words or thinking about an answer, you have a moment in which to run or strike. This is particularly useful when confronted with multiple assailants. Ask something completely unexpected, like "What time is it?" or something really odd, like "What was Gandhi's batting average?" Cognitive dissonance is powerful. During the opponent's momentary confusion, you will have an opportunity to act. Similarly, if you can hit an aggressor while he is talking, it takes about half a second for him to switch gears mentally from communicating to fighting.

Kane saw a great example of this when he watched a police officer confront an assault suspect. The guy was shirtless in unseasonably cold weather and appeared to be drunk and/or on drugs. The suspect wasn't particularly argumentative, but he was not cooperative either. Despite the officer's questions about what he was doing and repeated orders to show his hands, he refused to respond and continued to keep his right hand in his pocket. Assuming he had a weapon, the officer suddenly shot one hand up to grab the guy's throat, lifted him upward a few inches to break his balance, and then stepped forward to use his entire body weight to slam the suspect onto the ground. Continuing in one smooth motion, he rolled the guy over and calmly said, "Don't resist, don't resist," while simultaneously placing him in handcuffs.

This trick worked flawlessly because the officer made his move without any obvious pause or preparation, striking in midsentence while the suspect was focused on his words rather than his actions. It was a great example of disguising the "tell." Once the guy was on the ground, the officer's orders not to resist not only kept the guy from struggling but also helped witnesses understand that he was not using excessive force, which could prove crucial should witnesses be called to testify in court.

For better or worse, your words truly are a weapon. The challenge is that they can hurt you just as easily as they can harm your adversary. Use them wisely.

Don't Get Hung Up on Name-Calling

Name-calling means nothing unless you give it value. It should be meaningless when it comes to fighting, save as a distraction to use against the other guy. We have all heard the same old expletives and insults so many times that they no longer have significance.

Unfortunately, it is not always easy to keep this perspective. Calling one's masculinity into question, for example, is designed to attack the deepest part of one's psyche. And it can work if you let it. Name-calling is a trick designed to knock you off your mental equilibrium. When you are mad, you are not in total control. When you are not in control, you're vulnerable.

Think of the classic movie scene where the hero hits the villain in the face. The villain just smiles, and maybe spits out some blood, and continues the fight. Name-calling is like the first punch in a fight; it is meant to put you off balance. If you respond to the name-calling, you have reeled from the first punch. Worse yet, if the other guy can goad you into throwing the first blow, you become the bad guy. Now he has free rein to tee off on you with impunity. After all, he's defending himself from your aggression.

Do your best not to respond to insults. By understanding that they're not truth but merely a way to get at you, they can become a punch you will choose not to receive.

It is important to note that the intense emotional response that words cause may be harder to ignore than injuries caused by weapons. For example, you can be wounded in combat with an adversary and never know it until after the dust settles, suddenly discovering that you've been stabbed, shot, or badly mangled once the adrenaline wears off and the pain kicks in. There are hundreds of cases in which soldiers on the battlefield suddenly discovered that their legs had been blown off when they tried to stand up after a firefight.

Calm, reasoned responses will help you win in a fight, yet if you lose your cool because of what someone has said, your technique gets thrown out of whack. Fighting when enraged makes you a bit stronger and faster but far less skilled. Against a competent opponent, your rage will get you busted up quickly.

If You Have Made a Mistake, Apologize

Imagine this scenario: You walk out of the restroom at your neighborhood bar and accidentally smack into another guy, spilling his beer. He gets pissed, calls you a derogatory name, and takes a swing at you. There are a few different ways this can end without your being injured: You can walk away, he can walk away, he can be dragged away on a stretcher, or he can be carried away in a box. All these options accomplish your goal of not being hurt, but some are better than others.

What might happen if you can evade his punch and say something along the lines of, "Whoa! I'm sorry, I didn't see you there.

Let me buy you a new one"? Conversely, what will certainly happen if you immediately begin to fight back?

You can often tell when someone is in the wrong by how he reacts. Anyone who is unwilling to admit that he made a mistake is eventually going to take the argument to a personal level. Rather than continuing to debate the merits of the disagreement, he suddenly changes tactics and insults start to fly. At that point, the conflict is no longer about the mistake; it is about dominance, control, and saving face. Violence will often follow.

If you are in error about something, it is usually best to admit it. Remember, honesty is a better way to de-escalate a bad situation than lying or stubbornly refusing to acknowledge a wrong.

Your life and physical well-being are worth fighting for, while your possessions and self-esteem are not. Unfortunately, however, when you apologize to an aggressive person, it will often be seen as weakness. You may very well be verbally attacked for saying that you are sorry, hence feel compelled to fight. Don't fall into that trap.

The apology rarely goes like this:

You say, "I'm sorry! That was my mistake. I was wrong. It won't happen again." The other guy replies, "Thank you! It is rare that someone is willing to admit when they are wrong. You're a real stand-up guy. I hope you have a good evening."

It is more likely to work this way:

You say, "Sorry, man, my fault." He replies, "Damn right it is!" You respond, "Yes, it was, sorry." And then you walk away. Before you get too far you hear him retort, "F%&king pussy!"

Your goal is not to fight. If you walk away, your goal will be achieved. There can be no fight unless he follows you. Expect to get a couple more verbal jabs as you leave, though, maybe something challenging your manhood or your sexuality. Either way, leave it alone. Go somewhere else and enjoy your evening.

Name-calling is never worth fighting over. If the other person challenges you in this way, it is because he wants to fight. He thinks he can win. If he follows you and subsequently attacks, you will be on the side of the angels when things go to court. More often than not, however, he's just trying to provoke you into making the first move, or establishing dominance, and will let you walk away.

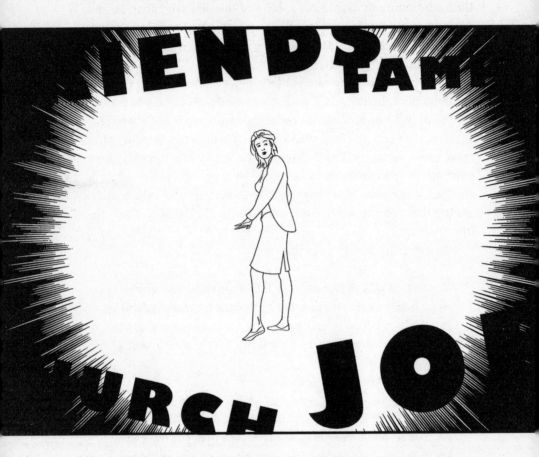

The reason for this type of aggression should not be important to you. You don't care if the guy who challenged you had a bad childhood, was molested, or is just out with his crew of friends for the evening and wants to look like a tough guy. You don't need a fight. You don't want a fight. Chances are, if he's spoiling for a fight, you are already outnumbered or overpowered, or something else is stacked in the other guy's favor, not yours. Maybe he's got a weapon palmed and is ready and able to use it.

Don't find out how he has stacked the deck unless he forces you to. Be the bigger man and walk away. After all, the tougher you truly are, the less you should feel a need to prove it. If you have made a mistake, apologize and be done with it.

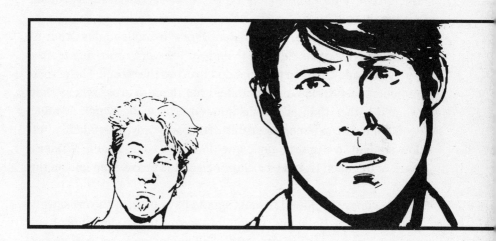

Make Sure Your Intentions Are Clear and Understandable

If you are in a face-off with someone, your adversary has made the decision that you are an easy mark. Before he hits you, however, you might still be able to make him rethink that decision. It is still a negotiation until someone gets hit. Consequently, words are critical before fists start to fly. They can still de-escalate the confrontation or even stop it dead in its tracks.

"Don't f%&k with me!" is an old, tired expression that means nothing. The bad guy has certainly heard that before and most likely beat down the last guy who said it. Snarling something along the lines of "I am going to rape you when I am done with you," on the other hand, changes the picture.*

You need to have the physicality and demeanor to make it a convincing threat, but your adversary will certainly get the message. Your intention—making him realize that he's picking on the wrong guy—is clear and understandable. You are scary. By breaking the conventions of what is expected, you seize the high ground, militarily speaking.

Wilder remembers an incident from his college days that illuminates this point. Several friends of his were returning from a party on campus when they needed to cross the street. The combination of inebriation and cockiness led them to cross where they wanted rather than at the designated crosswalk, which at night would have been a more sensible choice. As they jaywalked, a fellow student in a sports car came down the road. Seeing Wilder's pack of drunken friends, he slammed on his brakes and laid on the horn.

Of course, Wilder's friends should have been at the crosswalk waiting for the light, but the guy in the sports car should not have been going over the speed limit. And really, was the horn necessary? Add to it the driver had his girlfriend in the car, so he undoubtedly felt that he needed to yell an obscenity or two at the drunken horde to look good in her eyes. Everybody was in the wrong and alcohol was involved, a dangerous combination.

Here's the real mistake: The guy was in a car so he felt he was safe. We all have directed some kind of remark to another driver that we would never say in line at the bank, because we're in a car that physically separates us from the other person. However, this was a sports car with the top down. Even if the top had not been open, windows are surprisingly easy to break. At this point, the driver had made his intention clear—a verbal and public admonishment of the drunken goofballs who stepped into his path.

---

* If you are going to make a threat this extreme, you'd damn well better not lose the fight, though. A threat of male rape after a fight could very easily sway a jury that your opponent's killing you afterward was an act of blind and justified fear. Sometimes a solution for one part of the conflict complicates all the others. Choose your words wisely.

Wilder's friend Chris, on the other hand, had another intention. He turned, placed his foot on the front bumper of the sports car, hopped up onto the hood, and with two quick, and very heavy, hood-denting steps prepared to kick in the windshield. He stated, loudly and clearly, "What the f%&k is wrong with you, a*&hole!"

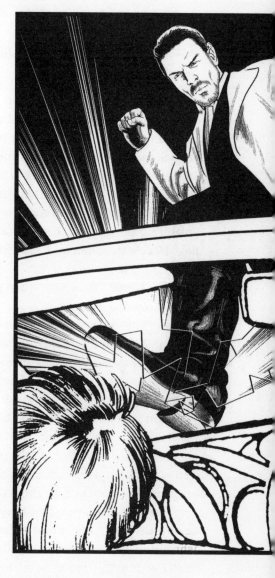

Now, this vignette is not about right and wrong, or even about justification; it is about making your intentions clear. The driver's intent had been to shame these guys in front of his girlfriend for crossing incorrectly. Wilder's friend's intention was equally clear—to do violence to the driver. He demonstrated his capacity for violence for all to see, metaphorically going from zero to sixty in the blink of an eye. Not exactly a response that the driver expected. If he were willing to do what he just did, what else would he be capable of?

Sure, everybody was in the wrong at several levels. What if the driver had pulled a gun? Would Wilder's friend have been able to stop it? Would you? Would you be willing to risk it? Hopefully not. Regardless, the point here is that Chris was willing to take that risk. He was willing to show just how far he was able to go. The message he conveyed by crushing a car hood was clear— "You're next!"

If you wish to preclude violence verbally or through some act, make sure that you are communicating what you intend and that you understand the risks in acting on that intention as well.

Changing the Context Can De-escalate a Bad Situation

An angry or aggressive person may simply want to vent his outrage. In many instances, you can do much good by calmly listening to him as he rants, all the while preparing yourself to act if attacked, of course. Interjecting a few choice words as necessary to help him see the situation in a new light can be very beneficial. Changing the context in this fashion can often de-escalate a bad situation by giving the other guy an out, some face-saving way of handling things that he was unable to see before.

Here's an example: Kane stopped at an Arco station to get gas on his way home from work. Their price was roughly ten cents per gallon cheaper than any other gas station in the area, so it was very crowded. Because the automated kiosks by the pumps were not working, he had to go into the store, wait in line to prepay, and then go back out to fill his tank. After doing so, he had to go back into the store to retrieve a couple of dollars in change.

As he approached the door, he could hear shouting coming from inside. Two women were arguing with the clerk. As Kane stood in line, he could not help but hear their dispute over the next several minutes. The women claimed to have given the clerk $22 to prepay and asserted that he put the money on the wrong pump. They said that they had received no gas and wanted him to either restart the pump or give them their money back.

He first countered that they had not paid him. The argument continued, with the women restating their claim and the clerk changing his response several times, such as stating that they had told him the wrong pump number and that it was not his fault if someone else pumped gas on their dime. As the argument escalated, one of the women in line behind Kane went outside to call the police. Several others simply left without buying anything. Everyone was very uncomfortable.

The distraught women were dressed in dirty coveralls, had some sort of ID badges that Kane could not read clipped to their waists, and were very buff. He imagined that they worked as mechanics, maintenance workers, or something similar and had just gotten off work. Neither was a small person; they were both close to six feet in height. The clerk was shorter and skinnier than either woman. He had a heavy accent and was a little hard to understand, especially when he raised his voice. Eventually, as one of the women called the clerk a liar for the umpteenth time, he retorted that she was a "fat, uppity bitch." This, as you would probably expect, did not go over too well.

The insulted woman went stiff, then spun on her heel and headed toward the door while her friend continued to argue with the clerk. As she turned past Kane, he got a good look at her face and jumped several notches up the threat index scale. The last time he had seen that "thousand-yard stare," the guy left a building, then returned a short time later with a gun.* Fearing something similar, he decided that he had better do something about it.

As she left, Kane noticed that she used her right hand to open the door and that she wore a watch on her left wrist, so he assumed

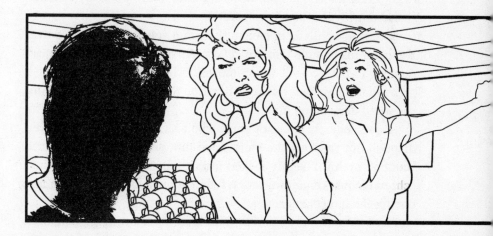

---

* Kane wisely bailed before that guy returned, reading about the aftermath the next day in the local paper.

that she was right-handed. He followed her out as she stalked toward her car. She was not moving fast, so he easily caught up a dozen feet past the door. Figuring that she was not armed (yet), he took a position a couple feet behind her left shoulder so he would have time to react if she did anything untoward.

Having positioned himself where he wanted to be, he calmly said, "You know, they have half a dozen video cameras in there. Your transaction must be on tape."

She froze in place but was not really processing what he said, so he repeated it again, adding, "All you need to do is have the manager review the tape to prove your story. There are cameras out here too, so they'll know that you didn't pump any gas." What he did not add was "And they'll record anything stupid you're about to do too," but she figured that out on her own as he intended.

She slowly said, "You're right, they do have cameras in there." She paused to think for a moment and then repeated more confidently, "Yeah, they do have cameras in there." As she did so, he could see the rage draining from her. She turned to face him and said eagerly, "They have cameras in there," once again, adding, "Thank you."

He replied, "No problem. You probably ought to explain that to your friend." She corrected him, telling him, "She's my cousin," then said, "Yeah, I'll talk to her."

While she pulled her cousin aside and began to calm her down, Kane got his change from the clerk. As the clerk handed him the money, he pointed out the cameras to him too. The clerk got a goofy look on his face as the realization that everything was being recorded dawned on him.

Kane honestly does not know who was telling the truth in this dispute, but the look the clerk gave him seemed to validate the women's claim. The guy looked guilty, something that Kane suspected from his changing story, frustration, and getting personal* during the interchange.

---

* Personalization is taking an argument to a personal level, such as the "fat, uppity bitch" comment from the salesclerk. He was no longer focused on what happened with the $22 but rather on the character of his accuser.

The interesting thing is that while the presence of a half a dozen highly visible cameras was obvious, no one in the dispute seemed to notice them. Pointing them out changed everyone's context. Kane will never know for sure if the angry woman was going for a weapon, but he's certain that he prevented something bad from happening when he intervened. He did not stick around to find out how it was resolved, though he did see a police car coming toward the place as he was driving away.

It is possible to de-escalate a tense situation by changing the context. Kane did not choose sides or make himself a target, but rather pointed out an essential fact that everyone had overlooked. This calmed things down long enough for rational thought to overrule emotion.

"That's f%&king b%$#sh*t," growled the tattooed, goateed guy at the bar, berating the waitress with a string of invective that could make a drunken sailor blush. The waitress walked away but Wilder, who overheard the argument, could not. From his table across the room he felt compelled to say, "You're a tough guy."

The tattooed guy leaned back in his chair, turned his head toward Wilder, and snarled, "You wanna see how tough?" He crossed his muscular arms across his broad chest and glared dead-eyed across the room, waiting for a response.

Now Wilder had a decision to make. Would he escalate the issue to a fight? He belatedly realized that he had foolishly thought he was going to point out the other guy's rudeness and get an apology, while the other guy was ready to fight and looking for an excuse to do it.

Realizing that he needed to send a different message, Wilder looked into the other guy's eyes, gave a nod toward the football game playing on the bar's TV, and asked, "Who do you like, Vikings or Lions?" The tattooed guy smirked and shifted his gaze back up at the television without saying another word. Wilder had answered his question; his query about the football game stated, in essence, "No. I really don't want to find out how tough you are."

Does such a response make Wilder a wimp? Was he a loser for not wanting to fight for the waitress's honor? After all, he's a black belt in three different martial arts. Shouldn't he have taught this rude guy a lesson in manners? Of course not. He understood the consequences of such actions and chose the better part of valor. Win or lose, if it came to physical blows, Wilder would have been in serious trouble.

Would it have been worth being sued for everything he owned, accumulating thousands of dollars in legal fees while having his reputation dragged through the mud, or becoming crippled, maimed, or even killed over a few rude words? Definitely not!

Know what is worth fighting for and what is not. Unless your life or the life of another is on the line, it's almost always best to swallow your pride and walk away. Live to fight another day.

CHAPTER FOUR

Live to Fight Another Day

Little Things Are Often Important

See the knife clip in the right front pocket of his blue jeans? Right there—you know he has a knife. Turning his right hip slightly away from you is a tiny little motion, yet it is going to get real significant in a moment. Once he turns a bit, you can no longer see that knife. Now you need to watch his right hand, yet he has dropped that back too. Suddenly you see his arm begin a slight upward movement. Is he innocently scratching an itch or pulling out that knife in order to gut you with it?

It all takes place in a fraction of a second—little time and tiny movements. Unfortunately, these little things can snowball into a serious crisis in a very short period of time too. What about the quiet guy in the corner? You're discussing politics, religion, or some other emotional topic with your buddies when you notice movement in your peripheral vision. That guy in the corner suddenly sits up straighter. As he gets up out of his chair, you notice that he has lowered his shoulders and slowed his breathing. He then moves purposefully toward you with a serious look on his face. Does he need to take a pee real bad or is he about to attack?

Little things that become important also include environmental considerations such as terrain, weather conditions, escape routes, sources of cover or concealment, bystanders, impromptu weapons, and so on—another reason why situational awareness is so important. If you want to take best advantage of these factors, pay attention to the details you're given before trouble starts. You'll be far too busy defending yourself afterward.

Terrain, for example, can help or hinder you. If you can take the high ground in an uneven environment such as a hill, stairwell, or pile of debris, it becomes much more difficult for your opponent to reach you or prevent your escape. Spilled blood, oil, or foodstuffs, loose gravel, wet grass or leaves, mud, and other hazardous conditions may affect your footing. If you are aware of these surroundings, you can adjust your stance, find a stable place, or maneuver your opponent onto slippery ground to gain an advantage.

Similarly, weather conditions may help or hurt. It is hard to fight with the sun in your eyes. Heat, humidity, and dehydration can sap your stamina, increasing the urgency of ending a fight quickly. Conversely, it is tough to grapple in powdery snow, icy conditions, or pouring rain, making it easier to get away if you can control your balance, posture, and speed.

Little things are particularly important when it comes to weapons. If you do not realize that the other guy is armed, you are in serious trouble. It's more than just that, though: Bullets that miss or pass through their target continue to travel downrange, potentially striking innocent bystanders. Impromptu weapons like bottles, bricks, boards, rocks, pool cues, fire extinguishers, flashlights, hammers, and wrenches might be lying around in close proximity for you or your adversary to pick up and use. Self-defense sprays such as Mace or pepper spray don't work very well in windy, rainy, or enclosed areas, where they might dissipate or blow back in your face. Grappling with a Mace-covered adversary can be problematic; that stuff is both extremely slick and highly irritating to your eyes, nose, and throat.

Be wary of bystanders too. Unless they are people whose job it is to get involved, such as bouncers, security personnel, or law enforcement officers, you really don't know what they might do. They may be inclined to help you, but they could just as easily ignore your plight in favor of their own safety or for fear of legal repercussions. Or they may be inclined to hurt you, especially if they are friends with the other guy. Knowing whether or not people hanging around the scene are part of the same group can be important. Even if bystanders do not get directly involved, witnesses may be called upon to testify to your actions in court, so in addition to fighting off your adversary, you need to be cognizant of how witnesses will perceive what you choose to do. Once again, details count.

Restrain Impassioned Friends

You know him affectionately as "No-Shirt Guy"—you know, the one who's always bouncing up and down, screaming, and generally making an ass of himself in the stands while you watch the game. A few beers and some harsh words later, and predictably, your buddy is fighting with some other fan. Now, instead of enjoying yourself, you're trying to drag him off the other guy, calm things down, and make sure no one is seriously hurt, when suddenly the police arrive. A few hours later, you are bailing him out of jail. Again.

Or perhaps you know him by some other name, such as "Chip on His Shoulder Guy." Regardless, it's always the mouthy friend who gets things going, isn't it? These guys come in many different flavors—small and mouthy, big and arrogant, crazy, or just plain dumb. Don't let his big fat mouth write a check that you need to cash.

Here's a good example. It was late in the third quarter of an exciting college football game where Kane was working security. Fans from both teams had packed the stands near the end zone. Throughout the game, there had been the typical taunts and insults you might expect in that sort of environment, but nothing serious had occurred, despite the fact that one group of home-team fans from the northeast side kept running in front of the visitor fan section on

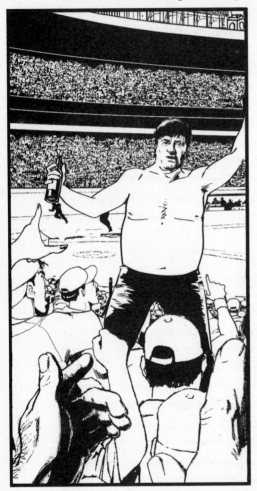

the southeast side and bopping around in a little victory dance with each big play or touchdown that was scored.

As illicit alcohol flowed and tempers ran hot, Kane and his crew took increasingly strict measures to keep the rowdy fans apart. They drew an imaginary line between the two sections, telling rowdies on both sides that so long as they stuck to their own section, they could rabble-rouse to their hearts' content. Cross the line to taunt the other team's fans, however, and they'd be thrown out of the stadium. Guess who the first person was to cross the line? Why, No-Shirt Guy, of course.

He got in an argument with the security guard who tried to prevent him from reaching the opposing fans. No-Shirt's friends, slightly smarter or more sober, were trying to hold him back, without success. Kane, realizing from a few yards away what was about to happen, grabbed a few additional guards, radioed the police, and moved to intervene.

Unfortunately, by the time he got there, the security guy already had a bloody nose and No-Shirt was beating his chest in glee, doing his best Tarzan imitation, with the injured guard lying at his feet. He even elbowed one of his friends, who was trying unsuc-cessfully to hold him back, cracking him hard enough in the cheek to make his teeth snap together.

The police showed up at the same time. Since they had seen everything, they were able to take direct action. Seconds later, No-Shirt Guy was in handcuffs. While the police led him off to jail, Kane escorted his friends out of the stadium, took their tickets, and ordered the gate guards not to let them back in. Despite the fact that they had not directly participated in the altercation, they got thrown out. They'd already been warned twice and the third time was the charm.

Collectively, they missed one of the most exciting games of the year, an affair that was decided by a clutch field goal in the waning seconds of the first overtime period. No-Shirt Guy wrote a check that his friends had to cash along with him. While they were not injured and, fortunately, did not have to cool their heels along with him in jail, they still paid a price. It could have been far worse and, if they keep hanging out with him, undoubtedly will be in the future. Restrain impassioned friends. If they insist on behaving immaturely, find new ones.

When It Comes to Violence, Girlfriends Can Be Helpful . . . but Generally Not

Some girlfriends think it's sexy for you to fight over them. They will go out of their way to set up situations where you can prove your manhood by doing so. This is ancient, tribal thinking. There was a time in the world when that type of behavior was essential to choosing a mate. The biggest and strongest male ensured her survival in a hunter-gatherer or early agrarian society.

This behavior has no place in the modern world. If your girl-friend thinks that getting you to bash some guy upside the head is cool, you are with the wrong woman. You need to take a deep look at where that behavior is coming from and why you are attracted to it, and consider how it is going to get you in trouble. And then you need to leave.

"Baby, that guy over there just called me a bitch," she might say. "Go over there and demand an apology from him!" Are you going to walk over to that big, bald, tattooed guy with the pool cue in his hand, who is glaring at you with an unblinking eye? Most likely not. At least not if you are smart. Does the scenario change if he is a short guy with a pocket protector and thick glasses held together with athletic tape? It probably does, but it shouldn't.

In 1984, four young men accosted Bernhard Goetz on a New York subway. A self-employed electrical repairman, Goetz could be described as a classic nerd. Whatever version of the story you may have heard, despite the guilt or innocence of all involved, four people were shot in about one and a half seconds during that encounter.

Goetz, who carried a concealed weapon, had practiced speed-shooting extensively. His gun was more than an equalizer, it gave him the advantage. How many other nerds might you run across who carry a weapon? Knife, gun, pool cue, baseball bat, or beer bottle, it makes no difference—dead is dead, maimed is maimed, whatever the cause.

If you are thinking "fight" and the other guy is thinking "combat," you are in for a world of hurt. If your girlfriend wants you to fight for her honor, get another girlfriend. Our recommendation is the same when the genders are reversed. This guy is trouble; you need to look real hard at what is happening to you. Dump him now and find someone else to hang out with.

Don't Claim Your Turf

Claiming your turf is about as tribal an act as you can commit. And it's sure to lead to trouble.

Wilder heard a story about a twenty-two-year-old, David, who had gotten into a bar fight with another guy. When the fight was broken up, the other guy was eighty-sixed from the establishment. As he was leaving, shouting and challenges ensued, and threats were made, yet David chose to stay in the bar for the rest of the evening. He was having fun with his friends. It was his turf, he'd claimed it, and he wasn't about to give it up. He did not want to go home until closing time.

As he headed to his car, he found himself confronted by the other guy. This time he had a gun. Seconds later, David was dead in the dirt from a bullet to his brain. For good measure, the other guy put one in his eye too. Then he fled the country. A promising life cut short with no possibility of justice.

It's only common sense; if you get in a fight and win, you need to leave soon afterward so that you cannot be found again that night. Revenge happens—a lot. It is not your turf; you don't live there. No matter how much you like the place, it's still just a bar. If you really want to keep drinking, go find another establishment a long way away. Or, better yet, call it a night.

A turf mentality means that someone has to win and someone else must lose. It almost guarantees violence, because the other guy has no face-saving way to back down. He leaves or you make him leave; there's no in-between. That's unnecessary, juvenile, and dangerous.

If you are mature, you don't fight unless you have to. When your life or that of a loved one is on the line, when you face grave bodily injury or death without fighting, then you pour it on with all you've got. When you don't have to fight, however, you walk away. It's the smart, mature thing to do.

Maturity means being confident in who you are. Taunts, threats, and name-calling will not injure your ego badly enough to make you feel a need to lash out. There is no good reason to stake your turf. Turf is for gangs to fight over because it is their livelihood. That's where they deal drugs, sell guns, manage prostitutes, and commit other crimes to earn their living. Turf means nothing to you, at least not if you are smart.

Darn Near Everybody Has a Knife . . . and It Changes Everything in a Fight

Do a little drill for the next few days. Carefully look at people's pants pockets, especially guys' pockets. Look for the bulges of pocketknives or of the metal clips used for securing folding knives. Look at belts for holsters for multi-tools, fixed blades, and other types of knives. Once you start looking, you'll see knives everywhere. That's because 70 percent of the adult male population in the United States carries one on a regular basis.

After the tragedy of 9/11, stadium security has dramatically increased across the country. Nevertheless, walking through security at Qwest Field (the Seahawks' stadium in Seattle), we spotted twenty-two people illegally carrying knives before they got to their seats. It's not that these people were a bunch of hardened criminals, mind you, but rather that knives are so common and carried so habitually that people bring them darn near everywhere. Even the heightened security had not stopped them, because there were no metal detectors and no pat-down searches, only bag checks and visual inspections.

Knives are supposed to be tools, but more often than not, they are seen as weapons. If you are looking at young men when you do the drill, you will see more knives; older men will have fewer; women fewer still. Young men often carry a knife as a security blanket, a subtle way of saying, "I am dangerous." And they are.

There are two kinds of people who carry knives—those who know what they are doing and those who don't. Most people fall into the latter category, but it doesn't really matter. Skilled or unskilled, nearly any person can cripple or kill you with any knife they choose to wield.

We have a friend named Jeff who works as an emergency room physician. In addition to being a doctor, he is an accomplished martial artist and military veteran. Wilder once asked him, "Have you ever looked at a person bleeding on your operating table and thought to yourself, 'The guy who did this really knew what he was doing'?" Dr. Jeff answered, "No. Violence is violence."

You need to remember that statement. The end result of contact with a knife, whether in the hands of a pro or the hands of a punk, is the same. It's all bad.

From time to time, Kane teaches a seminar on the realities of knife fighting. It is primarily designed to scare the crap out of people who don't fully appreciate what a blade can do to a human being. Among other things, he shares autopsy photos of unfortunates who did not learn that important lesson.

While the graphic pictures have made more than one student lose his lunch, the demonstration that really hits home goes like this: To show just how dangerous a knife is, Kane hangs a large hunk of meat—something that comes on the bone, such as a leg of lamb—from a rope. He then takes a folding knife with a legal* 2.5-inch blade and makes three cuts—a horizontal slash, a vertical slash, and a stab. After slicing up the meat, he whips out a measuring tape to show the damage. He can consistently make gashes in the meat that are five to six inches long and two inches deep. It's quite easy to do with a sharp knife; most students can duplicate that feat. He can also reliably strike the bone with the stab, even when it takes two to four inches of compression to do so. The noise of the blade hitting the bone is particularly chilling. After showing what a legal-length blade can do, he duplicates the experiment with a larger weapon. That can get really scary.

If you are thinking feet and fists, only to discover a knife in the middle of a fight, you are more than likely doomed. The stark reality is that most victims of weapon attacks do not recognize the severity of the threat in time to react properly. Imi Sde-Or, the founder of the martial art Krav Maga, wrote, "Victims who survived a violent confrontation against a knife-wielding assailant consistently reported that they were completely unaware of the existence of the weapon until after they had suffered stab or slash wounds. In essence, these survivors of edged-weapon attacks

---

* In most jurisdictions.

state that they believed they were engaged in some sort of fist-fight; only later, after sustaining injuries, did they realize that the assailant was armed."

You really needn't think "knife" at all; any old weapon will do. Wilder knows a guy who was hit so hard in the face with a beer bottle that the bottle shattered. Unlike in Hollywood movies, real bottles are pretty tough to break. That strike not only knocked him out, but he still bears the scars today. That fight ended right then and there—one blow, one weapon. Done.

Near everybody has a knife and it changes everything in a fight. Consider this carefully before you escalate a confrontation.

Gangs Are Not Your Friend

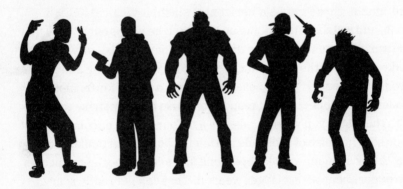

Gangs are groups of people who share a group name and identity, interact among themselves to the exclusion of others, claim a territory, create a climate of fear and intimidation within their domain, communicate in a unique style, wear distinctive clothing, and engage in criminal or antisocial activities on a regular basis. We're not talking about a Little League team here. Gang members frequently utilize tattoos, scars, or cigarette burns to announce their affiliation. These markings are usually obvious, seen on the arms and/or chest, but can also be discreet, such as a tattoo on the inside of the lower lip. Even their vehicles may be distinctive, with lowered frames, neon, excessive chrome, or tinted windows.

Gang members hold three things preeminent—respect, reputation, and revenge. If you cross a gang member in any manner, things will get ugly fast. Even looking at one with the wrong facial expression can get you seriously hurt or killed. Imagine a gang-banger's reaction to a more obvious sign of disrespect, such as a derogatory comment or physical blow.

Gang membership crosses all racial, ethnic, social, and economic lines. There are Asian gangs, black gangs, white gangs, Hispanic gangs, skinhead gangs, outlaw motorcycle gangs, and so on. Both male and female gang members instigate violence, carry weapons, deal drugs, participate in crimes, and take leadership roles within the organizations. They carry the marks of violence with pride, comparing knife scars, bullet wounds, burns, and various disfigurements to prove how tough they are and augment their reputations. Gangs get involved in everything from drug trafficking and manufacture to robbery, auto theft, carjacking, burglary, felonious assault, rape, murder, kidnapping, weapons trafficking, arson, prostitution, fraud, identity theft, vandalism, money laundering, extortion, and human trafficking.

According to the U.S. Department of Justice's official law enforcement tallies, there are more than 21,500 active youth gangs in the United States, with more than 800,000 members. These gang members account for roughly 10 percent of all violent crimes as well as 10 percent of homicides in the country. This does not include prison gangs, motorcycle gangs, or adult gangs, which would drive these percentages much higher. Furthermore, according to the Bureau of Justice Statistics, less than half of all gang-related crimes are reported to the police.

While some youths seek gang affiliation to make up for parental abuse or neglect at home, others simply crave the lifestyle, which is popularized in music, videos, movies, and television shows. Regardless of how they get involved, the gang becomes the member's surrogate family. If you mess with one gang member, you have messed with all of them. This can result in anything from a severe beat-down to a homicide.

However much respect you might feel you want or deserve, the average gang member craves it tenfold. Gangbangers will do everything they can to disrespect others while propping up themselves. Graffiti, hand signs, verbal challenges, stare-downs, and physical assaults are common in gang culture. While it is typically targeted at rival gang members, innocent civilians can easily become targets and/or get caught in the middle. New gang members are frequently required to commit a violent crime to cement their place.

Reputation is so important that gangbangers will even brag to the police, admitting crimes or even making them up on occasion in order to boost their status. For example, when a twenty-five-year-old gang member was arrested after a 2005 club fight in which a thirty-six-year-old victim was beaten to death, he told the responding officers, "I got good elbows. People don't know about my elbows." He later pled guilty to negligent homicide when it was determined that an elbow to the head had caused the victim's fatal trauma.

Gangbangers tend to live in the moment, doing whatever they feel like without regard to consequences. Many do not expect to live past the age of twenty-five. That can seem like a pretty long time if you get initiated into the gang at the age of thirteen or fourteen.

Revenge is a huge deal with gangs. If a gang member feels disrespected or thinks that his reputation has been harmed, retribution will certainly follow. No assault or insult can be left unanswered, no matter how small.

Wearing the wrong colors, traveling in the wrong area, or gazing with an unsuitable expression can bring about the same type of murderous retribution, such as a rape, murder, or physical assault. While this vengeance is often swift, that is not always the case. Asian gangs, for example, sometimes talk about the "hundred-year revenge," patiently waiting for the right opportunity to strike.

Listen to the Subtle (and Not-So-Subtle) Warnings You Get

While awareness is important on the street, don't turn your brain off at home. According to the Bureau of Justice Statistics, more than half of all homicides are committed by someone known to the victim. That means that your wife or husband, girlfriend or boyfriend, sister or brother, friend, relative, or acquaintance might just do you in someday.

Case in point: "She took a fishing knife out of his tackle box and stabbed him seven times in the chest. Killed him," Wilder's business partner, Rick, told him over the phone. "What, you mean your painter, Jeff?" Wilder asked. "Yep," Rick replied. "Stabbed him last night while he slept."

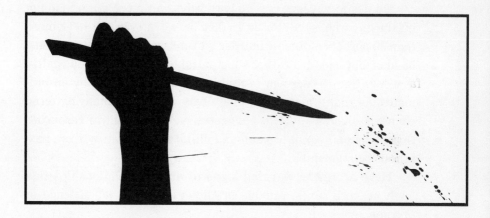

Jeff was a good employee. He was always on time, had a talent for painting cars, and loved the outdoors. Jeff's girlfriend, on the other hand, was wild. She was a real knockout but had little control over her emotions. In fact, the police had been to their home several times, especially on the weekends. She had even been sentenced to jail for assaulting him before.

Sadly, Jeff never stood a chance that night. While he peacefully slept, she went into his tackle box and pulled out a boning knife.

The blade was sharp and light with a long, tapered point and a keen edge. She crept into their bedroom, held the knife high over his chest, and thrust it downward into his heart with both hands. Then she pulled it out and slammed it in again . . . and again, and again, and again, and again, and then once more for good measure. And then she left the house.

Everybody who had ever met Jeff liked him. He was pleasant, easy to know, and honest. Anybody who met the two of them, however, had difficulty understanding their relationship. While everyone was saddened by what had happened, it didn't really take anyone all that much by surprise. In fact, not too long before the incident, someone had joked, "I hope she's really good in bed, man, because you know she's gonna do you in one day." All the hints were there, the warnings loud and clear, yet Jeff did not heed any of them. Now he's dead.

Domestic violence can go both ways, yet more often than not it's the guy who is the abuser. In fact, between 1976 and 2004, more than 30 percent of female murder victims were killed by their husband or boyfriend, a rather substantial number when you realize that less than 10 percent of male victims were killed by an intimate over that same period. That's why we have so many battered women's shelters, victim advocates, and community resources that focus on helping women and children move away from hazardous relationships.

Here are some warning signs of abusive relationships that apply to both sexes, reliable predictors of eventual violence or murder.

■ Your partner frequently yells at you, reprimands you, or demeans you in public. You have cause to fear his/her temper or are concerned about what kind of mood he or she is in on a regular basis.

■ Your partner isolates you, prevents you from getting or keeping a job, keeps you from seeing friends or family, or otherwise alienates your friends or family so that they feel uncomfortable being around that person. This is another method of cutting you from the herd, eliminating your support group.

■ Your partner keeps you from leaving your house or apartment from time to time, or conversely, occasionally locks you out of your home.

■ Your partner threatens to hurt or kill you, your children, your family, your friends, or your pets. All such threats, even ones made in jest, should be taken seriously.

■ Your partner hits, slaps, pushes, or shoves you, pulls your hair, or inflicts unwanted physical injury on you in any way, even during sex. The first time your significant other strikes you should be the last. Screaming and yelling might be tolerated on occasion, but physical abuse never should be.

■ Your partner exhibits extreme jealousy, checking in on you frequently, following you around or hiring someone else to do so, going through your mail, or installing monitoring programs on your computer. He or she becomes angry when you talk to or look at people of the opposite gender even when you have a legitimate reason for doing so.

One of the most important things a domestic abuse victim can do is get away from the perpetrator before things get worse. It is easy to rationalize or procrastinate, hoping that things will get better. Most of the time, however, they won't.

It can be tough to leave, but you must do it. Don't be embarrassed to death. Leave. There are plenty of resources to help you do the right thing and keep yourself safe. In most communities, there are both government and private agencies that can help you work through these issues, providing relocation, temporary housing, and medical assistance, and attending to other needs as appropriate.

There are some very interesting differences between men and women when it comes to fighting that can also become important in dysfunctional relationships. For the most part, men have "hot" rage. If they're going to lash out violently, it will be in the heat of anger. Women, on the other hand, tend to have "cold" rage. They're the ones who will take revenge long after the incident that inflamed them has passed, quite possibly after you've forgotten all about the argument, indiscretion, or whatever it was that occurred.

Listen to all the little warnings you get. Intimates can be just as hazardous to your health and well-being as strangers. Little hints can become bigger hints, small behaviors turning into larger ones. Pay attention and be safe.

CHAPTER FIVE

Food for Thought— You Will Get Hurt

As an eleven-year-old, Wilder and his friend Kim had gone down the hill toward the river to visit with a bum who had been camping out in the area. Wilder remembers standing there wide-eyed in wonderment as the old bum and intermittent jailbird explained how to put a sharpened screwdriver or toothbrush into an unsuspecting fellow inmate. "You stick 'em in the butt, right about here," he said. "That way the leg doesn't work so well and he can't run from you."

You may be thinking "fistfight," but that doesn't necessarily mean that the other guy is too. Knives, guns, bludgeons, beer bottles, and a host of other nasty tools may be in your adversary's arsenal. Think about that old jailbird's advice. It's chilling to think that he was counseling children on how to ambush someone in a fashion that ensured that the victim couldn't escape and they'd be able to kill him.

Whenever you fight, you are almost certainly going to get hurt, even if you don't run up against a psychotic foe. It's unavoidable if the battle lasts more than a few seconds. The real question is not if, but rather how badly, you will get hurt. If he's armed and you're not, the damage will almost certainly be severe. If he's bigger, faster, or stronger than you are, or he's got friends who join in, it's all bad. Remember, if he's attacking, he thinks he can win and is probably cheating in some way in order to do so.

Take this example: Most young men carry pocketknives these days. Many are willing to use them on you, either because they don't fully appreciate the consequences of their actions or, in some cases, because they are too furious to care. Then again, they may just be sociopaths like that old jailbird.

Knives are great tools, yet they automatically bump the encounter up from simple assault to aggravated assault or possibly murder. Use one on another human being without just cause and you'll spend a whole lot of time in prison, yet your average street punk isn't thinking that far ahead. He's reacting to the emotions of the situation, paying attention solely to the encounter he's in, right here, right now. In other words, all he cares about is defeating you, no matter how he has to go about doing it.

The vast majority of people who carry a knife have never used it as anything other than a tool for slicing fruit, opening envelopes, cutting up boxes, or similar routine endeavors. They have never hurt another human being with their blade. Unfortunately, they don't need any experience, special skills, or extraordinary intelligence to hurt someone badly with that knife. Heck, most any sharp object will do.

Think for a moment about the type of person it takes to want to ambush you with his knife. Premeditated attacks are worse than unhampered rage because knives are intimate weapons. That means that if you're facing the pointy end, the guy holding it either hates you with a white-hot passion or is totally out of his mind with fury and/or terror.

There is no reasoning with someone who is prepared to become drenched in your blood and viscera, to smell your bowels as they release, and to hear your cries for help as they fade to whimpers of pain and finally to the rattling gurgle of your last breath. If you are facing someone like this, he is willing to cut you as many times as it takes, to stab you as deep and as often as necessary to finish the job he has in mind. That kind of guy is real damn scary, be he a big brawny biker or skinny little computer geek. The blade makes them both deadly.

Fighting should be avoided whenever possible, because you cannot predict the chaos and mayhem that come along with it. If a knife or other weapon enters the fight, experience says that you are not very likely to see it before you have already been hurt. Badly.

It's hard for many people to visualize dying in a fight. Because of this, the threat of death isn't really much of a deterrent for most young men. Visualize instead spending the rest of your life maimed, crippled, or grossly disfigured, confined to a bed or a wheelchair. Think about all the things you'll never do and the places you'll never see in such a condition.

Although all violence is bad, armed assaults are far more dangerous to the victim than unarmed ones. Ordinary citizens are victimized an average of 1,773,000 times per year by weapon-wielding thugs in the United States alone. While crimes of nonlethal violence committed with or without weapons are about equally likely to result in victim injury, armed assaults are 3.5 times more likely than unarmed encounters to result in serious damage to the victim, such as broken bones, internal injuries, loss of consciousness, or similar trauma resulting in extended hospitalization. Worse still, 96 percent of all homicides involve some type of weapon.

Because you are going to get hurt, it is prudent to end the fight as quickly as possible to minimize the damage. This means that if you cannot avoid fighting altogether, your initial response needs to place you in control of the momentum. You need to keep from getting hit, stop the other guy from continuing to strike, and do it in as few moves as possible.

Once you have dealt with the immediate threat, your next move needs to cross him up, destroy his balance, or knock him on his ass. If he's got a weapon, your response should be, if not fatal, at least severely disabling.

DURING A VIOLENT ENCOUNTER

> Lotus seeds
> Jump every which way
> As they wish.
> —SOSEN (1694-1776)[3]

Unfortunately, there are instances when you have no choice but to fight and others where it is prudent to do so. We're going to give you some principles that can keep you safe, but no book can substitute for professional hands-on training when it comes to handling violence. If you are interested in learning how to defend yourself effectively, we suggest you seriously consider taking martial arts classes.

Fighting should never be your first choice, but sometimes it's your only option to keep yourself or someone you care about safe. In addition to learning some solid fighting techniques, you will discover some important principles that help you understand when you can legally get away with going physical. Unfortunately, countervailing force is not a yes/no equation. What you can and cannot do in the eyes of the law can be highly nuanced. Consequently, this section identifies appropriate levels of force that you might be able to employ while keeping yourself out of jail whenever you have to get hands-on.

Two Types of Violence

To the uninitiated, all fights look pretty much the same. But that is only because most people don't know what they are seeing. Nuances apply, but in essence there are two different types of violence: social and predatory. In the former, you are fighting over a matter of face or status, while in the latter you are fighting for your life. You can't treat them the same way.

The intent when it comes to blows in a social violence situation is to affect your environment. In other words, you want to establish dominance, to "educate" somebody, to get him out of your territory, or whatever. There are virtually always witnesses, because you're seeking status from the outcome, either by beating the other guy down or by making him back off.

Predatory violence, on the other hand, is completely different from social disputes. Violence itself is the goal. To begin, there are usually no witnesses (unless the predator has made a mistake). While the pickpocket might operate in a crowd, the mugger, serial killer, rapist, or arsonist won't. The predator's goal is to take you by surprise. If he does his job right, the victim never sees it coming until it's too late.

It's relatively easy to de-escalate social violence, particularly if you're willing to lose face. Clever words can give the other guy a face-saving way out, alleviating the need to fight. Unfortunately, the very things that might de-escalate a social situation will trigger a predatory attack because they make you appear weak. It's only possible to de-escalate predatory violence by appearing to be too dangerous to attack. If you're alert, aware, prepared, in decent physical condition, and setting a verbal boundary, that's a major warning sign to the predator, who will generally move on to easier prey.

Pay attention to your environment. For either type of violence, awareness is your best defense. After all, if you see it coming, you can either leave before you have to fight or prepare yourself to respond effectively.

CHAPTER SIX

Use Only as Much Force as the Situation Warrants

During the escalation process, there are several force options for staving off violence: (1) presence, (2) voice, (3) empty-hand restraint, (4) nonlethal force, and, ultimately, (5) lethal force. This continuum is similar to the approach codified by many police departments. The first two levels can potentially prevent violence before it begins, the third may be used proactively as an opponent prepares to strike, and the last two take place after you have already been attacked.

This continuum of force should be applied sensibly to preserve your safety as the situation warrants. Exceeding a reasonable level of force may well turn a victim into a perpetrator in the eyes of the courts.

Justifiable self-defense is a victim's defense to a criminal and/ or civil charge. The legal rationale goes like this: If your intent was to defend yourself, then a reasonable person would only do so using reasonable force. Sounds a bit circular but it is very important. Using a higher level of force implies that you had intent to needlessly harm the other guy. This allows the perpetrator-turned-

"victim" to use your defensive actions against you, the victim-turned-"perpetrator." Even if a criminal prosecutor dismisses your actions, a civil court may not do so. Bad guys sue their victims all the time. They even win too. It just isn't right, yet it certainly happens in this litigious society.

On the other hand, if you are too slow to escalate your response, you'll get the worst of the encounter, which is trouble of a whole different kind. Your response needs to be just right.

[1]
Presence

If you are a trained martial artist or just a well-conditioned athlete, your presence alone can frequently de-escalate a dangerous situation. Carry yourself with confidence and be prepared to act. Predators who are good at sensing body language may back off simply because they can tell that you are prepared to act. Bad guys don't want to tangle with you if they think they are going to get hurt in the process.

[2]
Voice

Use your verbal skills and tone of voice to talk an aggressor out of attacking you or otherwise get him to back down. Even when you cannot de-escalate a pending conflict through verbal skills, you may still be able to use your words as a psychological weapon to momentarily confuse or disrupt an opponent, giving yourself an opportunity to act. Your voice is a very important weapon in your self-defense arsenal. Don't forget to use it. Furthermore, be wary when the other guy tries to do the same thing back to you.

[3]
Empty-Hand Restraint

Restrain, disarm, and control techniques can be employed to keep an aggressor from hurting you and/or themselves until law enforcement professionals arrive. You will generally want to respond with a slightly greater degree of force than is used against you. But pulling a weapon on an unarmed attacker, for example, almost always makes you the bad guy.

Beware of things that *look* violent, like headlocks, chokes, etc. Pins, locks, arm bars, and similar control techniques are preferable if you can apply them safely and effectively. Be very cautious of going to the ground unless you are absolutely sure that your attacker acted alone and does not have friends who might take advantage of your vulnerability to attack, though.

Pinning or holding down the drunken uncle at a family gathering might work very effectively, while the same tactics used on an adversary in a crowded bar will almost certainly not. If you do use a restraint technique, try to hold the other guy facedown so that he has less chance of fighting free. Sports like judo require that you pin your opponent faceup, giving him a sporting chance, something that's bound to go poorly on the street.

[4]
Nonlethal Force

Nonlethal force includes striking, kicking, and a whole bunch of other martial arts techniques that cause damage to your opponent. Such strikes should be aimed at nonvital areas of the body. An elbow or knee to the gut is unlikely to kill your adversary, while the very same blow to his head could easily result in serious injuries, brain damage, or even death. Certain weapons such as pepper spray or Tasers can also be used for nonlethal force or restraint applications. Law enforcement and military professionals have an even wider array of nonlethal weapons (for example, water cannons, stun grenades, tear gas) to choose from than civilians do.

If restraint techniques do not work or will put you in danger because your assailant is armed or much bigger than you are, or there is more than one of them, you may have to escalate directly to this level should other options fail. Hit-and-run tactics such as kicking the knee or stomping the foot may slow your adversary down sufficiently to let you get away without needing to seriously damage him.

[5]
Lethal Force

Lethal force includes both martial applications to vital areas of the body (temple, throat, solar plexus, etc.) and deployment of weapons such as knives, guns, bludgeons, and the like. This level should be avoided unless there is no other way to escape a violent encounter unscathed. Your life must truly be at stake for you to use lethal force. And once you apply force that can kill someone, the fight will very likely only end when one of you is dead. You must be mentally and physically prepared to do whatever it takes to survive.

Is It Really Better to Be Judged by Twelve than Carried by Six?

Some self-defense experts throw around the phrase "It's better to be judged by twelve than carried by six." We do not advocate that sentiment, because we feel that it trivializes the seriousness of violent confrontations. Never forget that if you are found guilty in a jury trial, you will be spending a whole lot of time in a confined environment with unpredictable, dangerous neighbors who may be less than friendly when you interact with them. Even if you don't go to prison, you could lose your job, suffer consequences in your family and community, etc.

Bad things can happen when you fight for your life, but that doesn't mean that you shouldn't fight for everything you're worth if it gets to that point. Under no circumstances should you let fear of legal consequences keep you from living through a violent encounter, particularly against an armed assailant. If you don't survive, everything else is meaningless.

CHAPTER SEVEN

Four Techniques You Can Use in a Fight

You don't need to be a master martial artist or seasoned combat veteran to survive a street fight. It helps, of course, but it's not a requirement. You do, however, need to have a few solid techniques you can draw upon, stuff you can pull off when you're surging with adrenaline, scared witless, and really need to stop the other guy. There are three important yet very simple rules when it comes to self-defense:*

1. Don't get hit.

2. Stop him from continuing to attack you.

3. Always have a Plan B.

The first rule we've already described to you. "Don't get hit" is always sound advice. Previously we've discussed this rule in the context of awareness, avoidance, and de-escalation, but it's true for fighting techniques as well. If whatever you do doesn't

---

* The fourth rule not mentioned here is "Don't go to jail." We've already covered judicious use of force, so we won't rehash it again in this section.

keep you from getting hit, the rest doesn't matter all that much. Once you've been hurt by the other guy, it gets progressively tougher to fight back. Consequently, you need to block, deflect, or evade his attack before you can do anything else. Sometimes that's done by preemptively striking, though more often than not it's by some sort of defensive movement. That's not ideal, but it's reality.

The second rule, "Stop him from continuing to attack you," is just as important. You can block, deflect, or evade all you like, but that won't end the fight. You need to perform a technique or combination of movements that incapacitate the other guy, persuade him to leave you alone and break off his attack, and/or facilitate your escape.

The goal is to ensure that he can no longer hurt you. The faster you can do that, the better; conversely, the longer the fight, the more likely you are to get hurt.

Winston Churchill wrote, "No matter how enmeshed a commander becomes in his plans, it is occasionally necessary to take the enemy into consideration." In other words, no matter how crafty you are, whatever you try is not necessarily going to work. The other guy is trying his damnedest to pound your face in, pulling out every dirty trick he can think of in an effort to mess you up. Whatever you attempt may knock him on his ass straightaway, but oftentimes it doesn't work out that way, so it's prudent to have a Plan B.

It's obvious that if you can pummel the other guy into submission, you win, but that's not your only option. If the other guy can't get close enough to reach you in the first place, he will not be able to strike. Controlling distance is important. It's very tough to fight if you can't see, so the eyes may be a viable target, at least in life-or-death encounters. If he is on the ground when you're still standing, you have a much better chance of getting away. Of course, you can always hit him . . . a lot. To this end, we suggest four things that you may wish to try in a fight.

- *Don't let him get close enough to touch you.*
- *Throw debris to distract or injure him.*

- *Attack his eyes.*
- *Strike with impetus.*

You've probably noticed that, with the exception of controlling distance, these are offensive techniques rather than defensive ones. While it's important to be able to block or deflect the other guy's attack, it's more important to take him out of the fight as quickly as possible. Our goal is not to turn you into the ultimate street fighter, but rather to give you a few options that you might be able to pull off without a whole lot of practice. If you really want to get good at the physical aspects of fighting, you are going to need to find a martial arts school and sign up for hands-on instruction.

Don't Let Him Get Close Enough to Touch You

Distance is crucial in a fight. If you are too far away, he can't strike you. If you are too close, the range limits the available weapons your attacker and you can use to fight each other. Combat begins at about ten or more feet from you. Positioning is initiated, openings are looked for, reactions and responses are judged. This entire process may take as little as one ten-thousandth of a second, as that is how long it takes for the brain to process information. Or it could take the better part of an evening.

Letting somebody get close to you is an invitation for a fight. And be careful after you think you've resolved a dispute and the guy comes in for a handshake. That handshake is an opportunity for him to get close, control one of your weapons and your balance, and give you a sucker punch. An arm around the shoulder is the same thing.

No matter what he asks, your answer should be no. If he is sincere in his attitude, he will shrug it off and go about his business. If not, he will take offense and escalate the situation again. His response tells you everything you need to know about how it was going to go down, so either way you are ahead.

Every situation is unique. In England and much of Europe, for example, you could be at risk from a head butt in a fight, whereas that type of attack is rarely seen in the United States, where a punch to the face is more common. Either way, your adversary must get close in order to reach you. It is critical, therefore, to maintain sufficient distance between yourself and a potential assailant to give yourself time to respond to whatever he tries to do.

An unarmed attacker poses a danger to you within about ten feet. For an attacker armed with a knife or bludgeoning object, this range is extended to a bare minimum of twenty-one feet. The bad guy can close that distance shockingly fast. A second or two is all he needs to move in and strike. While that may seem a rather lengthy separation, research has been conducted that validates this assertion. Sergeant Dennis Tueller of the Salt Lake City Police Department conducted a series of tests showing that people of various ages, weights, heights, and physical conditions could close a distance of twenty-one feet in an average time of 1.5 seconds, about as long as it takes a highly trained officer to draw a handgun and fire one or two aimed shots. Knowing that people who have been shot do not often fall down instantly, or otherwise stop dead in their tracks, Tueller concluded that a person armed with a blade or a blunt instrument at a range of twenty-one feet was a potentially lethal threat. In fact, it takes a fatally wounded person between ten and a hundred and twenty seconds to drop, so you must fire and then move off-line while expecting your attacker to continue his assault even after your bullets have hit him.

In training as well as in real-life encounters, police officers are frequently unable to draw their guns and fire a shot before being cut, sometimes fatally, by a knife-wielding opponent moving toward them from distances as great as twenty to thirty feet. It is reasonable to assert that the average civilian is somewhat less prepared for such encounters than the typical law enforcement professional.

Distance can help keep you safe even when your attacker has a firearm. Most gunfights take place at a distance of less than ten feet. In fact, according to FBI statistics, 95 percent of officer-involved shootings occur at less than twenty-one feet, with approximately 75 percent taking place at less than ten feet and a little over half at closer than five feet. The farther away the other guy is, the tougher it is for him to hit you. Further, you have a much better chance to escape to safety or dash toward some source of cover that can protect you.

Throw Debris to Distract or Injure Him

Throwing debris is really an extension of distance. It is not a stand-alone technique, but rather a facilitator that can keep the other guy back and help you escape. You can kick dust, throw rocks, hurl trash, swing garbage cans, or otherwise chuck stuff at the other guy to distract or potentially injure him. Don't throw your weapon if you have one, though. You're going to be giving up your best source of defense by throwing it away.

Here is a rough way to estimate your ability to throw an object and have a reasonable chance of hurting somebody; Wilder calls this the "baseball test." It was developed through rigorous threshold testing while he was at college. To do the test, march off about a quarter of the dormitory hallway floor, turn, and face the fire door at the end of the hall. Make sure no one else is around.

Using a baseball, not a softball, hurl the ball at the fire door at the end of the hall. If you can hit the door, good for you. If you can dent the door, in theory you have thrown hard enough to injure the other guy in a fight. Both accuracy and force are required. We're not actually advocating that you go out and damage someone else's property, but hurling a baseball at a door hard enough to make a dent really does indicate the kind of speed and accuracy necessary to injure someone with a thrown object. Since it's tough to actually injure, you're most likely going to use this tactic to distract.

Before you employ this tactic, however, identify your escape route. You need to know that before you do anything else. It doesn't do much good to throw things unless you can do it in the interest of providing an opportunity to escape. For our purposes, if it isn't nailed down, it is debris. Look around the space you are in right now to see what is available to you. Are the chairs too heavy? What about a couch? Dresser drawers? How about a silverware drawer full of pointy objects? Pictures on the walls, stuff in your pockets, objects on your desk, or whatever is lying around that you can get to quickly and is heavy enough to be some sort of threat but light enough to throw with some accuracy will do the trick.

Throw at the other guy's face. It's the most distracting and potentially damaging target. The weight and size of the debris may affect your accuracy, but it's important to target where you will get the most reaction. When you throw, move to the escape route at the same time. The debris will only give you a second or two, so you need to use it to your best advantage.

Attack His Eyes

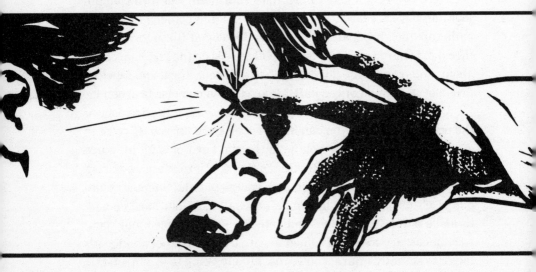

It's really tough to fight if you can't see. That makes the other guy's eyes a very important target in a legitimate self-defense scenario. Compared to all our other senses, eyesight is dominant. It's not only how we view the outside world but also how we acquire targets and defend ourselves against assaults.

When you have an opportunity to attack the eyes during a fight, the chance will only be there for an instant. If you're going to go for the shot, you've got to take advantage of that moment of opportunity. The thing about attacking the eyes is that it is similar to attacking the groin; there is a natural guarding reflex, even in unskilled fighters, that is difficult to get past.

Think back to the last time you were riding in a car and something hit the windshield. You instinctively flinched, didn't you? When the rock hit the windshield, your eyes closed, your shoulders lifted, your head went forward and down, and your hands came up. In essence, you tucked your head in like a turtle pulling its head into its shell. This reflex action protects the neck, eyes, and face. It gets as much flesh around the eyes as it can by squinting, making them well defended.

Knowing that the other guy is going to have this natural protection for his eyes means that there is a good chance you won't be successful the first time you try to strike him there. You need to be fast, well trained, and usually a little lucky to get his eyes on the first try. Assuming you are fast and/or lucky but not highly trained, you will need to keep trying until it works.

This is serious stuff. Not only can you cause horrific injuries with eye attacks, but also you let the other guy know that this is a very serious confrontation. If you attack his eyes and miss, you're really going to piss him off in a primal way, becoming the target of a lot more anger and violence than you might expect. Anything goes from that point on.

Anybody who wears glasses can relate to this. Have your glasses knocked off by another guy, even accidentally, and it pisses you off. It is personal, it is primal, and it's instantaneous. Even in an accident, it takes a certain amount of effort to control the instinctive reaction. This gives you a glimpse of the type of response you will elicit from a person when you attack his eyes.

So, while attacking the eyes can incapacitate an adversary, it can inflame him too. Consequently you need to know how to do it right. The best techniques use either your thumbs or fingers. Here's how to attack the eyes most effectively.

Thumbs

The thumb can be used as a wedge to displace the eyeball from the eye socket. This is done by placing your thumb against the inside of the bridge of his nose and pushing into the corner of his eye socket. Typically, you'll use your fingers as a guide alongside the guy's face. It works much better if you can support his head with your other hand or block it with a solid object such as a wall or the ground so that he cannot move his head back or twist away.

When shoved forcefully into the eye socket, your thumb works much like a wood-splitting wedge, displacing the eyeball. You don't have to fully pop the eye from the socket; simply stretching the optic nerve is excruciating painful. This makes the eye short out, for lack of a better phrase, causing blurred vision, disorientation, shock, and in some cases blindness, more than enough trauma to let you escape to safety in most cases. If you actually displace the eyeball, the disabling effect is even more severe.

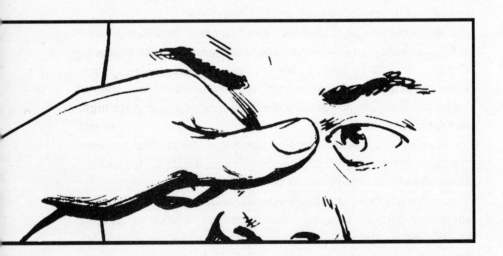

Fingers

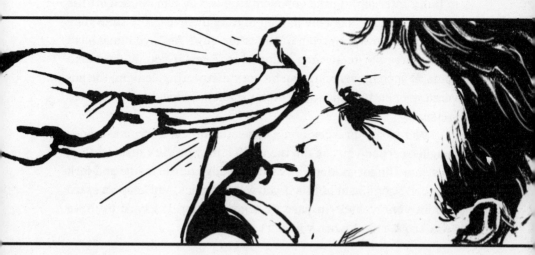

Raking the eyes is about damaging the cornea, the outer covering of the eye. Scratching the eye in this manner causes excessive tearing, light sensitivity, and pain. A vertical claw brought down the face from eyebrow to cheek will most likely fail. Moving your fingertips laterally across the eye, on the other hand, is likely to be much more successful.

This attack is done powerfully, more than once, and with resolve. The chances of failure without these three points are high. Attempting to put the fingertips into the eye is a strike better left to the skilled martial artist. It is fast and effective but can hurt your hand if you do it incorrectly. Everyone else should follow this method of horizontal raking.

In this example, we will use the left hand. Using an open hand, thrust your palm forward so that it smacks into the attacker's cheekbone. This bone will serve as an anchor and guide. Thrust the fingertips into the eye (the number of or which fingers is not important) and in a twisting motion, similar to the motion you'd use to take the lid off a jar of pickles, twist away from the attacker's nose toward his ear. Keep trying until it works.

If you are a trained martial artist, you almost certainly know how to do an open-hand chest block (for example, *hiki uke*). After initially intercepting the opponent's blow, you can bounce off his arm in a circular clawing motion to rake the eyes. Any time your open hand crosses in front of the other guy's face, you may have the opportunity to scratch at his eyes. Even if you do not make contact, such movements can be very distracting, leaving the adversary open to a follow-on attack such as a low kick or a knee strike.

If he wears prescription glasses (or in some circumstances sunglasses) and you can flip them off, it may be very disorienting. This same finger motion can catch the edge of the frame and jerk it free. Be cognizant of this if you wear glasses, and keep an extra pair in your vehicle in case they get broken. It's hard to drive away from a fight when you can't see.

Strike with Impetus

Sometimes hitting the other guy is your best tactic in a street fight. If you're a skilled martial artist, there are dozens of hand striking techniques that you might attempt, including fore-fist punches, standing-fist punches, sword-hand strikes, palm-heel strikes, hammer fist blows, back fist strikes, wrist strikes, swing strikes, uppercuts, and single-knuckle strikes, to name a few. Unless you have substantial skills, however, it is dangerous to hit a solid target with your closed fist. If your alignment is off, you will break your hand and/or damage your wrist. Wilder, who knows what he's doing, has broken his hand three times. It's not all that hard to do in a fight.

No matter how skilled you are (or are not), strikes work best when you catch your opponent by surprise, control distance and the direction of your blow, relax until the moment of contact, and strike ferociously and repeatedly until the conflict is over.

Surprise

As with any fighting application, if the other guy doesn't see it coming, you're much more likely to be successful. Be careful not to telegraph your blows. Each blow should suddenly explode, from wherever your starting point is, into your target as fast as possible with no warning. Avoid cocking your arm back, taking a sudden breath, tensing your neck, shoulders, or arms, widening your eyes, grinning, grimacing, or making any other inappropriate or unnecessary movement before each blow. The same thing applies to elbow strikes, kicks, and knee strikes as well. If you train in martial arts, practicing in front of a mirror can help eliminate these tells. Videotaping training sessions can also be a great way to objectively evaluate your performance and look for areas for improvement.

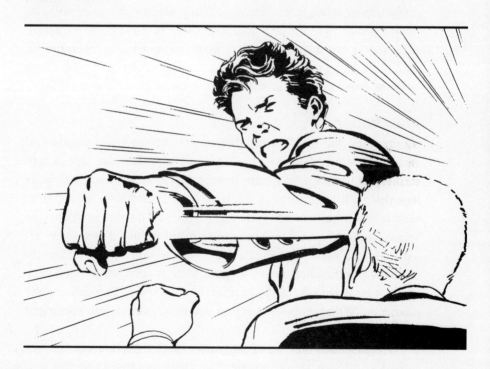

Distance

Ensure that you are close enough to strike before you throw a blow. That's often closer than you'd naturally think. If you have to roll your shoulder or lean forward, you are too far away. Whenever you have to stretch to reach the other guy, your alignment will be off, your blow will be slower, and your power will be significantly reduced. Worse still, it will be easy for your adversary to disrupt your balance and drive you into the ground. Furthermore, if you lock your elbow to get a few extra inches of reach, you can damage the joint as well.

Once you are in range, strike directly at the target, covering the shortest distance possible. Keep your elbow pointed downward and your arm as close to your side as possible. Hook punches, haymakers, and other wide-swinging blows take longer to reach your target than straight movements. They are much easier to spot, hence easier to block or avoid. The same thing applies for kicks. Unless you are skilled enough to disguise your intent, roundhouse and hook kicks are easier to block than more direct applications such as front kicks or joint kicks.

Relaxation

Controlling the mind is the difference between being good and being great. In Major League Baseball, a pitcher can have a ten-million-dollar arm, but pair it with a ten-dollar head and he is worthless. It's the same in fighting. If you are tense, letting your amped-up mind control your body, you will be slow and easy to block. It might sound counterintuitive, but it's not. Try it for yourself. Make a tight fist, lock all your muscles down hard, and try to throw a fast punch. Now try it again with an open hand. Flick your hand forward as fast as you can, as if you're trying to touch or poke someone. Which is faster? When you are relaxed, you can move much more swiftly.

Experienced martial artists know that relaxation does not require you to sacrifice power. The trick is tensing at the moment of impact, not before. Here's how it works: *Fa jing* means "explosive or vibrating power." It is sort of like a sneeze, a sudden unexpected movement that is very difficult to anticipate or block, followed by an instant of tension at the moment of impact. Both speed and relaxation are necessary to achieve *fa jing*. All strikes should be performed in this fashion. If you are relaxed until the moment of impact, your speed and power will be greatly increased. And, importantly, you will make it much harder for the other guy to defend himself from your blows.

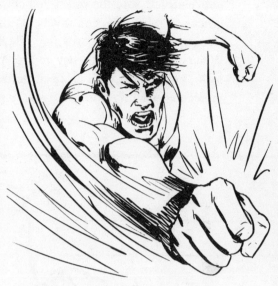

Ferocity

All things being equal, the guy who attacks with the most ferocity wins. Even if the other guy is a bit stronger or more skilled than you are, he's likely to disengage if he realizes he's bitten off more than he can chew. If you have no other choice but to fight, do so wholeheartedly. Your adversary should feel like he's run across a rabid wolverine wielding an industrial buzz saw. Strike fast, hard, and repeatedly until it's over and you can escape to safety. Throwing a single blow or short combination and dancing aside to see if it had any effect may work well in the tournament ring, but it's woefully inadequate on the street. Give it everything you're worth and don't stop until it's over.

Hand strikes, forearm strikes, elbow strikes, knee strikes, foot strikes, and head butts are common applications that can be successfully employed without too much training.

Hand Strikes

The hand is a great weapon in a fight. We've already mentioned that you don't want to hit a solid object with your knuckles unless you are very skilled, yet you don't need to make a fist to hurt the other guy. Palm-heel strikes, for example, can be very powerful yet relatively safe for you if you contact something hard like the other guy's jaw. You can thrust straight out with your open palm (for example, to the face) or slap sideways (for example, to the ear). When we teach children how to break boards for the first time, we have them strike with an open palm because they can generate much power with relative safety.

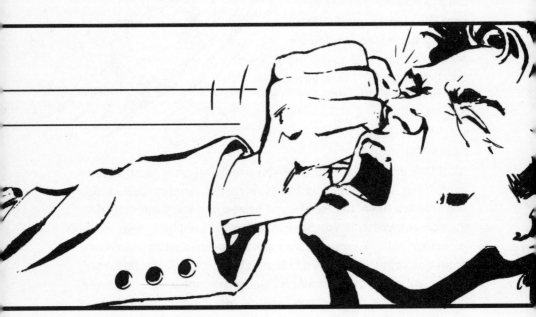

Rotate your hand upward and pull your fingers back so that you won't tangle them on anything. Aim so that you will hit with the meaty heel of your palm at the bottom. You can improve your power if you can get your body weight behind the blow too. The easiest way to do that is to step forward as you strike. Begin with the hand movement and then follow with the step. Your opponent will undoubtedly see the blow coming if you step first and then strike. The goal, however, is to land the blow at the same time you complete your step, adding impetus to the strike.

Another way to strike with reduced chances of injury to your hand is with a hammer fist blow. While this is done using a closed fist, you hit with the bottom of your hand rather than with your knuckles. This softer striking surface protects the hand yet can deliver solid power in your blows. You can strike downward (for example, to the face or nose) or sideways (for example, to the side of the head or temple).

There are dozens of other effective hand strikes, yet they require a fair amount of training to execute successfully and safely, so we won't go into detail here. If you do choose to punch with a closed fist, however, it's critical that you straighten your wrist and strike primarily with your first and second knuckles so that the line of power passes directly through the knuckles, traveling up your arm and into your body. If you connect with something solid like the other guy's jaw with a bent wrist or with your third and fourth knuckles, you can hurt yourself severely.

Forearm Strikes

A forearm smash can be extraordinarily powerful, though you need to be relatively close to an opponent to make it work. It looks like a basic head block in a striking art such as karate, yet it is designed to be offensive rather than primarily defensive in nature. Forearm blows work best when you rotate the hard ulna bone along the outside edge of your arm into the other guy, using the torque from your twisting movement to augment your upward force. Adding a forward step to magnify the blow with your body weight can be beneficial as well. Forearm strikes can also be executed sideways like a hammer fist blow, though that's usually intended as a defensive technique to block or deflect an opponent's punch.

Elbow Strikes

The elbow is a pretty hard bone, one of the hardest structures in the human body. Nature knows that you are very likely to land on your elbows in a fall, so the bone is very resilient. The elbow also serves as an excellent short-range weapon when you are too close to generate good power with your palm-heel strike or punch. You can create

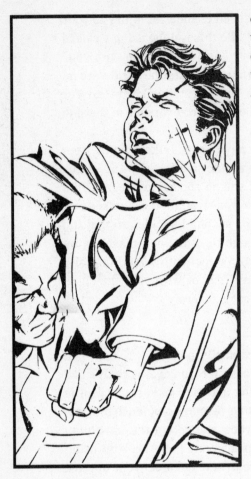

enormously powerful blows at very short distances using your elbows, one of the reasons this type of strike is favored in martial arts such as *muay Thai*.

You can strike upward (for example, to the solar plexus), downward (for example, to the head or neck if the other guy is bent over), or sideways (for example, to the ribs or head) with your elbow. You can strike directly behind you too. It is a very versatile weapon. It is also important to note that only the most skilled practitioners have the forethought and skill to use their elbows as weapons in most cases. The majority of people default to their closed fists in a fight, even when the distance is better suited to a shorter-range weapon such as the elbow. Consequently, elbow strikes can have an additional element of surprise when you use them on the street.

Knee Strikes

Your knee is much like your elbow. If you know how to joint-lock an arm, you know how to joint-lock a leg. If you know how to strike with your elbows, you also know how to use your knees. Once again, short range is key for knee strikes. If you are too far away, they do not work effectively.

Obviously, the groin is a default target, one that is often taught in women's self-defense classes. The challenge is that men are inherently good at protecting their genitals. Further, groin strikes rarely end a fight right away. Fortunately, there are alternatives you might choose.

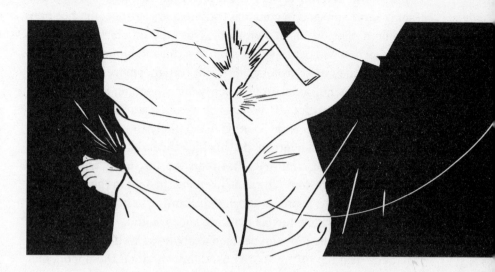

There is an easily accessible nerve bundle along the side of your thigh, about where your fingers touch if your hands are hanging down at your sides. That's a great place to hit with a knee strike if you're tangled up with a standing opponent. You can also knee-strike his chest or solar plexus if you are a skilled grappler or can find a way to get him off balance or bend him over first. For example, you can hook the back of his head with your hand, or cross your arms behind him to strike the back of his neck, and then pull him downward into your blow. Trying to use this technique without training can be dangerous, however, as it is fairly easy to become unbalanced when you strike that high with your knee.

If your adversary is on the ground, your knee can be used to strike his ribs too. This type of knee strike is often a precursor to grappling, as it is intensely painful and can flip your opponent onto his back or side. You can also strike to the head if he's down, of course, but that's very dangerous and challenging to justify in court unless he's armed. The knee can generate extraordinary power, so be cautious that you don't overdo things if you strike with it.

Foot Strikes

While most martial artists train barefoot, in today's world the foot is rarely unshod in combat. That means your boot or shoe can become a weapon in its own right. Not only do certain types of footwear make great striking surfaces (for example, a steel-toed boot), but they also protect your foot. Furthermore, proper foot positioning is not as critical when you're wearing shoes as it is when you are barefoot. If you're not wearing shoes and don't pull your toes back on a front kick, you are likely to jam them. Wearing sturdy shoes can let you do this kick incorrectly without hurting yourself. The similarity between the boxing glove and the shoe should not be lost. The shoe protects the foot in the same way the boxing glove protects the hand. Similarly, it often cushions and softens the blow too, as running shoes would.

The top of the foot can be used to strike as well as the toe and the heel. The top of the foot is used anywhere on the opponent's body. You will see the top of the foot and/or toe used on the face, usually when the opponent is down. If you are the person on the ground, be prepared to have incoming blows aimed at your face. The heel, or stomp kick, is also frequently used when the opponent is on the ground. It's simply a matter of downward versus sideways motion. Once again, be aware of the legal ramifications of using such techniques.

If you are going to kick the other guy in a fight, the safest place to aim is below his waist. Low kicks are faster, more direct, and harder to block than high ones. They also help you retain your balance. Front kicks, stomps, and side kicks are generally the easiest kicks for beginners to learn. You begin all of these kicks by forcefully lifting your knee as quickly as you can. The higher you lift your knee, within reason, the better. To do a front kick, swing your foot up and snap it forward. For a stomp kick, drive it back downward, leading with your heel. To do a side kick, rotate your hip and snap the kick out to the side. Good targets include the side of the knee, the middle of the thigh, the ankle, and the foot. You can also target the groin, though that's often challenging.

Head Butts

While head butts are very common throughout most of Europe, they are rarely seen in America. Perhaps this has something to do with the popularity of soccer, yet it really doesn't matter all that much why. What matters is that it works. Head butts can be used in very-close-quarters combat. The goal of the head butt is simple: forcefully striking one of the stronger bone architectures of your body onto a weaker area of your opponent's skull. This is usually done by driving your forehead into the occipital bone surrounding the other guy's eye, into his temple, or into his nose.

While the forehead is the most common striking surface for head butts, you can attack with all four sides of your head, connecting with the area as a sweatband would. Avoid hitting with "softer" areas such as your face, ear, or temple. It is imperative to note that the head butt is a body move, not a head move, especially when butting with the back of the head. If you strike solely with your head/neck, like nodding, you are quite likely to injure yourself, particularly if you miss. Use your whole body. Loren Christensen, a retired military policeman, civilian law enforcement

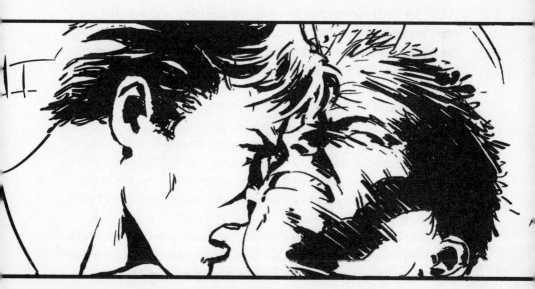

officer, and martial artist who has survived numerous violent confrontations, likes to call it "bowing with prejudice," an apt analogy.

Distance and surprise are critical for a successful head butt. Additionally, it's also important to note that you are momentarily blind when you perform the technique. Like trying to keep your eyes open during a sneeze, it's nearly impossible not to close your eyes on contact.

There are many ways to secure the other guy's hands and arms to keep him from interfering with your head butt, but that is not always necessary, particularly when you have the element of surprise on your side. An infamous example of this was when French soccer star Zinedine Zidane head butted Italian Marco Materazzi during the 2006 World Cup final. The two players exchanged heated words before Zidane began to walk away. Materazzi reportedly called Zidane's sister a whore, and Zidane turned around, made a run-up, and head butted Materazzi in the chest, knocking him to the ground. He was subsequently ejected from the game.

Combinations

While all of these techniques can be used in isolation, they are more effective when combined. The best combinations move along the body, going high-low-high or low-high-low to create openings by disrupting the opponent. They work because your adversary's head and hands will follow the pain when you strike him. His attention should shift to where he has been struck, particularly if he is not a trained fighter who has become desensitized to pain. Further, there is a natural physiological reaction that draws a person's hands toward the body part that hurts. This gives you a momentary advantage to strike an unguarded area, providing that your combinations flow smoothly and quickly in concert with one another.

For example, let's say that your adversary opens the fight with a punch to your midsection. One way to respond is by twisting to the side, evading, or shoulder blocking his punch and then immediately riposting with a palm-heel strike to his face. As he reels back from your hand strike, you can fairly easily stomp on his foot or ankle (or throw a low kick to his knee, depending on the angle of the opening). As his attention is drawn to the damaged limb, you can finish him off with a hammer fist blow to the face.

CHAPTER EIGHT

If You're Going to Hit Someone, Make It Count

If you have to hurt someone in a fight, you will need to target a vital area of his body, someplace that can be damaged relatively easily. Punching someone in the stomach, for example, may only piss him off, while striking him in the temple may render him unconscious. When executed correctly, vital-area attacks are extremely dangerous stuff. *Do not abuse this knowledge.* Such areas should only be forcefully attacked in true life-or-death situations from which you can only escape through violence.

Not every vital-area blow will have consequences such as we list here. It depends on how hard and accurately you strike, as well as what you hit with. Most people can deliver a pretty strong blow using their fists or unshod feet, while a severe blow requires help from some sort of solid object such as a baseball bat or steel-toed boot to increase the effectiveness of the strike. Highly skilled martial artists can often do extraordinary damage unaided.

It is important to note that individuals who are stimulated by adrenaline, fear, drugs, alcohol, or even sheer willpower may not be incapacitated from any blow that is not immediately physiologically disabling, even if mortally wounded. It is extraordinarily unusual to stop an adversary with a single blow.

VITAL AREAS CHART

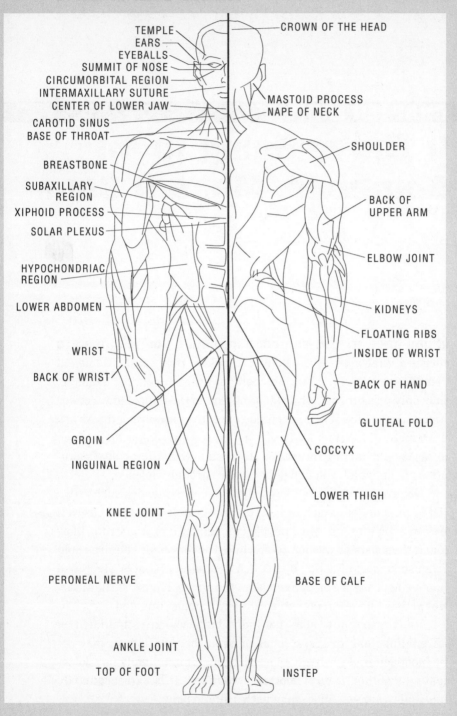

TEMPLE
EARS
EYEBALLS
SUMMIT OF NOSE
CIRCUMORBITAL REGION
INTERMAXILLARY SUTURE
CENTER OF LOWER JAW
CAROTID SINUS
BASE OF THROAT
BREASTBONE
SUBAXILLARY REGION
XIPHOID PROCESS
SOLAR PLEXUS
HYPOCHONDRIAC REGION
LOWER ABDOMEN
WRIST
BACK OF WRIST
GROIN
INGUINAL REGION
KNEE JOINT
PERONEAL NERVE
ANKLE JOINT
TOP OF FOOT

CROWN OF THE HEAD
MASTOID PROCESS
NAPE OF NECK
SHOULDER
BACK OF UPPER ARM
ELBOW JOINT
KIDNEYS
FLOATING RIBS
INSIDE OF WRIST
BACK OF HAND
GLUTEAL FOLD
COCCYX
LOWER THIGH
BASE OF CALF
INSTEP

VITAL AREA	DESCRIPTION
CROWN OF THE HEAD	Any blow to the head can be dangerous. A very strong blow to the crown of the head at the coronal suture could dislocate the frontal bone, causing severe damage to the motor regions of the brain, resulting in paralysis or death.
TEMPLE	The temple is the weakest structural area of the skull, where it flattens at the sides, about two finger widths back from each eye. The weakness exists because curves are architecturally much stronger than flat surfaces. The area is not only flat but thin and a confluence of suture lines—the temporal, sphenoid, frontal, and parietal bones—join here. Shock transmits through the skull most easily at these points. A strong blow to the temple can cause massive hemorrhaging of the meningeal artery, coma, and eventually death.
EARS	A concussive slap to the ears can cause pain, disorientation, and severe trauma to the eardrum, particularly if the hands are slightly cupped.
SUMMIT OF THE NOSE	A strong blow to the summit of the nose at the center of the forehead can shock the frontal lobes, causing unconsciousness, while a severe blow can cause death (though this has more to do with delivering force to the head than the susceptibility of the nose in particular).
CIRCUMORBITAL REGION	Located above and below the eyes. Hard strikes to this area can transmit shock to the frontal lobes of the brain, resulting in unconsciousness.
EYEBALLS	Eye strikes can cause anything from watering to blindness, depending on severity. When the adversary is standing, the eyes are usually attacked with a raking motion. When he is on the ground, such that his head can be immobilized, gouges or displacements may be used. This is frequently done by pressing the thumb or a finger into the side of the socket, which displaces and potentially ejects the eyeball. Excruciating pain and psychological trauma from this type of application usually render the victim unconscious. Permanent eye injuries may result.
INTERMAXIL-LARY SUTURE	Located just under the nose at the philtrum. The nerves are very close to the surface in this area, such that even a light blow can cause pain, watery eyes, and sensory disruption in most people. This sensitive area can also be used for control techniques when leveraged from behind (pushing in and up to manipulate the head/neck and control the spine). Smashing the middle of the face can be traumatic, interfering with respiration and causing airway bleeding and severe pain. Strong blows can transmit shock through the upper jawbones into the braincase, causing unconsciousness.

VITAL AREA	DESCRIPTION
CENTER OF THE LOWER JAW	A blow here transmits shock through the jaw into the inner ear, shaking the brain. Injuries can include broken teeth, dislocation of the jaw, whiplash, dizziness, or unconsciousness. Really severe blows, such as those from heavyweight weapons (for example, a baseball bat or sledgehammer) can dislocate the skull from the top of the spinal column, resulting in instant death. This spinal injury concept applies for the philtrum point as well.
MASTOID PROCESS	Located behind the ears at the sides of the neck. Blows to this area can affect the facial nerve, potentially causing pain and disorientation, though not necessarily enough to stop a determined adversary. This area is close to the brain stem, much like at the base of the skull. Neck "cranks" are often performed in this area as well.
NAPE OF THE NECK	Located at the third intervertebral space, the nape of the neck is the weakest point of the spinal column. A strong blow here can cause disorientation, unconsciousness, paralysis, or death, depending on severity.
CAROTID SINUS	Located at the side of the neck in front of the sternocleidomastoid muscle. A blow to this area can disrupt the baroreceptors, which regulate blood pressure flowing through the carotid artery into the brain. This can cause the heart rate to instantly drop, leading to disorientation or unconsciousness. This point is also used for strangulation techniques, in which applying pressure can cut off the blood flow, leading to unconsciousness or death.
BASE OF THE THROAT	The windpipe is very vulnerable just above the suprasternal notch. A blow or strangulation technique here can crush the cartilage of the trachea, leading to suffocation and death. A finger jab or push can elicit severe pain.
SUMMIT OF THE BREASTBONE	Located where the manubrium and sternum meet. A strong blow here can cause trauma to the heart, bronchus, lungs, thoracic nerves, and/or pulmonary arteries, leading to unconsciousness or death.
XIPHOID PROCESS	Located at the bottom of the rib cage in the middle of your chest, the cartilaginous extension of the lower part of the sternum. Striking this point, particularly with a rising blow, can bruise the heart, liver, and/or stomach, leading to unconsciousness or possibly even death.
SOLAR PLEXUS	Located just below the xiphoid process. A blow to this area can shock the diaphragm, rendering the recipient temporarily incapable of breathing. A powerful blow in this area can cause internal bleeding in the stomach and/or liver, leading to severe pain, unconsciousness, and even death.

VITAL AREA	DESCRIPTION
SUBAXILLARY REGION	Located below the armpits, approximately between the fifth and sixth ribs. A strong blow here, especially when performed with a single knuckle, can cause trauma to the lungs, disrupting breathing. This area can also be raked with a knuckle, causing considerable pain in many, but not all, people.
HYPOCHON-DRIAC REGION	Located between the seventh and eighth ribs, approximately one hand width below the solar plexus. A blow to the right side can severely damage the liver, causing internal bleeding. A blow to the left side can damage the stomach and/or spleen, once again causing internal bleeding. Either blow can have fatal consequences. Death is by hemorrhage, a slow process.
KIDNEYS	A strong blow to this region can cause internal bleeding, shock, and death. This area is frequently targeted using kicking techniques. Death is by hemorrhage, a slow process.
FLOATING RIBS	The eleventh and twelfth ribs are only attached at one end, making them more vulnerable than other ribs to breakage. A blow to the right side can damage the liver, while a blow to the left can damage the stomach and/or spleen.
LOWER ABDOMEN	Located approximately one inch below the navel. A strong downward blow to this area can damage the bladder and large intestine, causing extreme pain and loss of bladder control.
SHOULDER	This joint can be dislocated or hyperextended, rendering the arm unusable for combat.
BACK OF THE UPPER ARM	A strike to this area can affect the radial nerve, causing pain and weakness. A forceful rub in this area can affect the triple warmer (plexus of the radial, ulnar, and medial nerves), causing pain in many individuals and an involuntary rotation of the arm. This facilitates controlling techniques such as an arm bar.
ELBOW JOINT	A strike to the area about an inch above the elbow can affect the ulnar nerve (this area is sometimes referred to as the funny bone), causing pain and weakness. The joint can be dislocated or hyperextended, rendering the arm unusable for combat.
WRIST	The joint can be dislocated or hyperextended, resulting in temporary or permanent loss of use of the hand. The wrist is much harder to damage using joint manipulation techniques than the elbow or shoulder.

VITAL AREA	DESCRIPTION
INSIDE OF THE WRIST	Located where the pulse can be felt. A blow here can affect the median nerve, eliciting pain and weakness. Arteries are very close to the surface in this area, making them vulnerable to damage, especially from edged weapons.
BACK OF THE WRIST	A blow to the back of the wrist can affect the median nerve, eliciting pain and weakening the grip.
BACK OF THE HAND	The radial nerve is exposed between the thumb and index finger, and the radial and ulnar nerves meet between the knuckles of the middle and ring fingers. A sharp blow to these areas will cause additional pain and weakness, though a powerful strike to anywhere along the back of the hand can damage delicate bones. Digging the knuckles into the back of an opponent's hand can break his grip. The fingers may be attacked or manipulated too.
GROIN	Severe blows to this region can elicit pain, shock, nausea, vomiting, or unconsciousness in male victims. A firm grab to this area can also be incapacitating. Upward blows to the pelvic girdle of a female opponent can elicit similar results, though it takes a bit more force and accuracy.
COCCYX	Located at the base of the spine. Because the major nerves feeding the lower limbs originate in this sacral plexus region at the tailbone, a blow to this area can elicit severe pain. The coccyx is fairly easy to break with an upward strike, severely hampering an opponent's ability to move.
INGUINAL REGION	Located at the base of the spine. Because the major nerves feeding the lower limbs originate in this sacral plexus region at the tailbone, a blow to this area can elicit severe pain. The coccyx is fairly easy to break with an upward strike, severely hampering an opponent's ability to move.
GLUTEAL FOLD	Located just below the buttocks. The sciatic nerve, the largest in the body, is located here. A solid blow can cause cramping, loss of control of the leg, and pain throughout the hips and abdomen.
LATERAL PART OF THE LOWER THIGH	Lateral part of the lower thigh, about halfway down on the outside of the vastus lateralis (the large muscle). A blow here can cause pain and temporary paralysis of the thigh.
KNEE JOINT	One of the weakest areas of the human body when struck from the proper angle, this joint can be hyperextended or dislocated to disrupt balance and effectively take an opponent out of a fight.

VITAL AREA	DESCRIPTION
PERONEAL NERVE	Located at the center point of the tibia (shinbone) and fibula (bone on the outside of the leg). A blow delivered about two-thirds of the way down the shin can hit the peroneal nerve, bringing pain and weakening the leg.
BASE OF THE CALF	Blows to the inside of the lower leg at the base of the calf can cause pain and temporary paralysis of the leg muscles.
ANKLE JOINT	This joint may be hyperextended, dislocated, or crushed by a solid blow, causing severe pain, disabling an opponent's balance, and reducing his ability to move and fight.
INSTEP	A blow to the upper surface of the instep can damage the plantar and peroneal nerves, causing pain throughout the leg, hip, and abdomen, weakening the leg.
TOP OF THE FOOT	Like the hand, small bones in the foot are easily crushed, disabling an opponent's balance and reducing his ability to move and fight.

The vital areas listed above describe targets that are vulnerable to blunt force trauma, the type of damage typically meted out by the fist or foot, though occasionally by instruments such as baseball bats, batons, bricks, boots, and other solid objects. When it comes to bullets, ballistic performance (for example, penetration, expansion, energy transfer) and wound trauma (for example, level of physiological disruption) both affect stopping power, though shot placement is paramount. The only truly incapacitating targets are the brain and upper spinal cord, though wounds to the heart, major arteries, and lungs may prove severely disabling if not fatal in rather short order. Damage to the head or neck that does not disrupt the central nervous system, as well as hits to the arms, legs, stomach, and groin, may prove sufficiently painful to stop an attacker, though they are generally not immediately disabling and can be shrugged off by a committed adversary.

Common targets that have proven lethal or severely disabling with blade weapons include the heart, subclavian artery, stomach, brachial artery, radial artery, carotid artery, femoral artery, axillary artery, groin, and kidneys. Knife thrusts are generally more damaging than slashes, yet they also require you to move deeper into your opponent's target zone, where he can easily reach you with his weapon if he is similarly armed. Consequently, other frequent targets include the hands, wrists, and elbows, which may be cut at somewhat less risk of riposte. Such damage, while not immediately disabling, may convince an attacker to break off and retreat, though you certainly cannot count on that happening in every situation.

CHAPTER NINE
Down 'n' Dirty

In real life, it is critical to fight to the goal. Winning doesn't matter; it's not-losing that's paramount. Survive. At all costs. You are far better off not fighting, of course, but if you have to go physical, the shorter the fight means the lower your chances of getting seriously hurt. End it quickly. Your strategy must be to hit and run. Put him down and get the hell out of Dodge. In order to achieve this goal, you need to protect your centerline, move, and strike or defend simultaneously. This is sound advice for a fistfight, but it may be the only thing that can save your life when weapons are involved, so heed the lesson.

The following section is for readers who do not have an extensive background in martial arts. There are hundreds of styles, each with its own strategy and tactics. If you study one of them, use it. If not, this straightforward, effective advice can hold you in good stead without a lot of training when things get ugly on the street.

Protect Your Centerline

If you draw an imaginary line from the crown of your head down the front of your body, you will touch a majority of the vital areas of your body, things like your eyes, throat, solar plexus, and groin. These are areas that you really don't want someone to hit. A bladed stance like boxers use, with one foot forward and the body canted slightly, helps make it harder for the bad guy to reach your tender bits without reducing your range or striking power.

If you are right-handed, it typically feels more natural to lead with your left, and vice versa. Either way, the lead foot and hand should be the same. In other words, if your left hand is forward, your left leg should be too. Keep your lead hand high and forward to jab or deflect incoming blows and your trailing hand low and back near your side. Hunch slightly, raising your shoulders to protect your neck. Traditional martial artists won't consider this proper form, but it takes years to master more sophisticated methods.

Your weight should be evenly distributed on both feet so that you can easily move in any direction to attack or defend yourself. Stay upright and mobile, keeping your lead hand between you and your adversary. Strike, move, and strike some more as needed, until you can position yourself to escape to safety.

Stepping and Shifting

Stepping is how we travel long distances. We place one foot in front of the other, switching back to front as we walk, and do the same thing faster as we run. The challenge in a fight is that when we lift a foot to move, we become temporarily unbalanced unless sophisticated martial arts techniques are utilized. This means that, at certain times, shifting is more appropriate.

A shift is when we move forward or back but don't change the relative positions of our feet. In other words, if your left leg is back and right leg is forward and you take a step, they switch, whereas if you shift, the left is still back and the right forward after you finish the move. If you've ever watched Olympic fencing, you will see this type of thing a lot. It is not good for traveling long distances, but it does have its place in a fight, because there is a lower chance of tangling your feet and falling. Further, if you do it right, your center of gravity stays lower and you are harder to unbalance than when you step.

Combinations of stepping and shifting are used in most violent altercations. The trick is selecting the right movement for the tactical environment. This depends primarily upon how much distance you have to travel, what angle you must take, and what type of blow you want to deliver to your adversary. Shadowboxing in front of a mirror can help you get the hang of it.

Step Back and Strike

If the opponent takes the initiative faster than you can react, it is often useful to fade back and counterstrike. Timing and distance are important, so this technique is easier to perfect if you practice it with someone under the tutelage of a competent instructor. Nevertheless, this is something you can pull off without a lot of training, even when adrenalized, so long as you don't freeze up. Hit and run; that's the goal.

As the attacker advances, turn your body and step back so that your lead foot becomes your trailing foot while simultaneously throwing a blow. The lead hand moves back and down while the trailing hand whips out and up (or straight or down, depending on where you are aiming). Make sure you hit a vital area. You want to hurt the other guy, not piss him off. Your weight should be on the front foot when your blow connects, a natural response to taking the step that increases the effectiveness of your attack.

Done smoothly, this movement often takes your opponent by surprise, as it looks like you are retreating until suddenly he gets hit. When your blow connects, keep moving and throw another one if you are still in range. If things go well, you will have injured or stunned your adversary with one or two blows and positioned yourself to escape before he can reorient. This may be all it takes to get away.

Shift Forward and Strike

Sometimes you will want to take initiative and aggressively take the fight to an opponent. At close range, a shift can be the most effective way of accomplishing this. Begin by lifting your front foot and pushing off with your back leg, so that you lunge forward. Make sure that your legs stay roughly shoulder width apart and don't cross each other. If your stance gets too narrow, you are likely to lose your balance as you move. Don't hop either; this should be a smooth, low shift. Land your weight on your front foot and strike with the lead hand simultaneously (same side).

This is an explosive movement that takes advantage of your body weight to add impetus to your blow. Be sure to keep your elbow down; this helps connect the arm with the rest of your body. If your elbow drifts up or out, much of the force will be lost when you strike. Hitting with your whole body does a lot more damage than striking with just your arm.

Shift Back and Strike

If the other guy is coming in hot and heavy, you can still utilize a shifting technique to maintain proper fighting distance while counterstriking. It is almost the exact opposite of a forward-shift-and-strike technique.

Lift your back foot and push off from the front, lunging backward. Once again, maintain roughly shoulder width separation between your legs so that your stance doesn't get too narrow. As your back foot lands, strike with the lead hand. Once again, the lead hand and foot are on the same side.

This can be a much weaker blow than a forward shift, but if your adversary is barreling into you, then his momentum will increase the power of your strike. Keep your elbow down to connect your arm with your body. This not only ensures maximum damage from your blow but also helps ensure that your adversary's momentum doesn't bowl you over.

Slapping and Deflecting

Blocking is one of the most common misnomers in martial arts. The word *"uke"* in Japanese, commonly translated as "block," really means "to receive." That's a good mind-set in a fight. You don't want to stop the opponent's force so much as redirect it so that it will not harm you. And, importantly, you want to do it in a way that either hurts him or makes it easy for you to take him out with your next movement. Hit and run.

Slapping with an open hand is much faster than striking with a closed fist, especially for people without a lot of martial arts experience. While it is possible to simply cover up, using a motion that looks much like combing your hair to protect your head, by way of example, more aggressive defenses work better. Generally you will use your lead hand to do this.

Begin by guarding the centerline, holding your lead hand directly in front of your chest. From there you can flip your hand either upward and outward to protect your head, or in and down to protect your body. You can also deflect body shots side to side with minimal movement. Keep your elbow down while you slap upward or to the side, but let it rotate out as you slap downward. Don't worry about finesse; simply slap the incoming threat with your open hand.

You don't need to stop the blow, only move it aside just enough so that it doesn't hit you square on. Glancing blows are okay; they hurt but don't damage unless a weapon is in play.

The closer to the opponent you connect, the easier it is to deflect his strike. Try this: Have a friend hold a fist out in front of your face. Using your open hand, push his fist aside until it misses your head. Pay attention to how far you have to move it. Now do it again, but this time reach out to his elbow or a little higher on his arm toward his shoulder. How far do you need to push this time? It's a lot shorter, huh?

Use this concept. Reach out and slap the incoming arm to defend yourself, ignoring your adversary's hand. The arm moves comparatively slower as the blow begins, so reach out a ways toward your opponent too. This makes it easier to perform the maneuver and you don't need to deflect his arm as much in order to be safe. Immediately counterstrike so that he can't simply reorient and hit you again.

Slapping and Striking

Slapping and striking is virtually identical to slapping and deflecting except that you bring the other arm into play as well. As you defend yourself with your lead arm, counterstrike with your trailing hand.

If you can simultaneously shift diagonally to one side away from the blow, so much the better. In that fashion you can clear distance, making it harder for the opponent to reach you, yet also position yourself to strike him more easily. This takes practice, but it's really slick when you pull it off properly.

Striking to Disrupt

Striking to disrupt and disrupting to strike are very effective ways of breaking through the other guy's defenses. If you try to punch him in the face, for example, odds are pretty good that he will block it. Even untrained individuals are instinctively good at protecting their heads. We cover up our "soft bits" instinctually. Stomping on his foot or kicking his ankle first, however, causes his head and hands to follow the pain. He involuntarily looks down and flinches inward. This usually opens up the head shot. So you strike his foot, disrupting his stance and concentration, and then you use the disruption to gain the opportunity to attack his head.

In this fashion, you can work the other guy's body—striking to disrupt, and then using the temporary disruption for an even better strike. Attacks to the feet, knees, or ankles; slaps to the ears; and assaults to the hands, wrists, or elbows are all disruptive strikes that are much easier to achieve than starting off with the core, where all his vital areas are. It's really tough to get there directly.

With a good disruption, you can follow up with shots to his eyes, throat, solar plexus, groin, and other painful, vital targets.

Kick and Run

Kicking can be hard to do in a fight because it's easy to lose your balance if you are not highly skilled, but you can still pull it off if you keep things simple, straightforward, and low.

Begin by slightly bending the knee of your plant leg—the one you'll be standing on when you kick—and then forcefully lift your other knee straight up as fast and explosively as you can. If you are very close to your opponent, you will actually connect with the knee strike, but if he is farther away, you will need to use your foot or shin as the striking surface. Regardless of distance, that explosive knee lift is necessary.

Once you've lifted your knee, you will need to lash out with your foot. Stay low, aiming at the opponent's groin or lower. For an upward or forward shot, bring your foot up in an arc. Hit with the ball of your shod foot unless you have extensive training; barefoot is for professionals. If you're wearing boots, you can hit with the toe too. Alternately, you can strike out to the side or stomp downward. The knee, ankle, and foot make excellent targets because they are relatively easy to damage and harder to instinctively protect than the groin. In the flurry of battle, your adversary is likely not even going to see the kick coming, particularly if you strike toward his face with your hand first.

Once you connect, pull your foot back immediately so that it can't be captured by your opponent. Think "knee up, out, back." The faster you strike, return, and get your foot back onto the ground, the better. When your foot is in the air you are vulnerable. The combination of pain and surprise from your kick should give you an opportunity to escape to safety. After all, he can't chase you if he can't run.

CHAPTER TEN

Seven Mistakes to Avoid in a Fight

Real fighting on the street is nothing like practice in the dojo. When it's real, the consequences are real too. Your body knows this even if your mind does not. Adrenaline surges through your system, making you faster, tougher, and more resilient. It helps you survive yet robs you of fine motor control and higher thought processes at the same time. Your animal brain (amygdala) rears up and takes control, making it hard to respond, plan, or think your actions through. Consequently, you need to keep things simple and straightforward in order to be effective.

You must employ techniques that do not require fine motor coordination or complicated thought. These applications must also cause serious damage if you want to stop a determined aggressor who, like yourself, is also hopped up on adrenaline. Last, but not least, the techniques you choose cannot take very long to execute. John Wayne–style roundhouse punches, high kicks, and the like take far too long to deliver when compared to other techniques.

Because it is hard not to telegraph these types of big movements, they are easier for the other guy to see, hence easier for him to counter or block. This is bad not only because it doesn't work very well, but also because the longer the fight lasts, the better the chances that you will get hurt in the process. It is much better to use low kicks, straight punches, and other applications that hit hard, fast, and immediately.

To this end, we suggest seven things you should remember in a fight.

- *Don't kick above the waist.*
- *Don't play "tank."*
- *Don't hit with a closed fist . . . unless you've got skills.*
- *Don't forget to use your mouth too.*
- *Don't play the other guy's game.*
- *Don't use the wrong technique for the situation.*
- *Don't go to the ground.*

Don't Kick Above the Waist

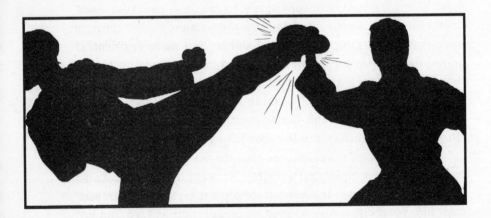

Funny things happen when you work stadium security. Way back when Kane was a green belt in karate, he had occasion to attempt to throw a patron out of the stadium for rowdy behavior. That sort of thing happened incessantly, yet this particular occasion was somewhat unique. Kane didn't know it at the time, but the other guy wasn't just disruptive and annoying; he was also a black belt in tae kwon do.

As they approached the gate, the rowdy fan suddenly wrapped his brain around what was happening and made up his mind that he wasn't going to leave quietly. Without warning, he suddenly spun and launched a lightning-fast roundhouse kick at Kane's head.

Sensing movement, Kane shifted slightly, instinctively scoop-blocking the kick. It's not that he was better or faster than the other guy—he most certainly was not—but the movement was so broad and telegraphed, and took so long to connect, that he was able to intercept the kick successfully. We're talking fractions of seconds here, yet it was enough, particularly since Kane had been practicing kick defenses over and over for a couple months prior to the incident while working on advancement requirements toward his next belt test. Because it was ingrained into his muscle memory, his body reacted without much conscious thought.

Once he had captured the other guy's leg, it was no effort at all to clamp it down onto his shoulder with both hands, holding it in place. He then started walking backward, dragging the other guy over to a police officer who was stationed at the gate nearby. The officer calmly watched Kane dragging the fan toward him, the former tough guy wincing in pain as his leg and groin were stretched and hopping along in an attempt to keep up without falling over. As the pair approached, the officer sardonically stated, "Hey, I can come back in a while if you'd like to hurt him some more." While Kane laughed, the other guy went a little pale.

The guy was underage, but he was not drunk, so he was off the hook for that one, but worse things were yet to come. The officer examined the rowdy's identification. Since he'd seen the kick and knew that most folks couldn't pull something like that off without practice, it was a logical question to ask about his training. The other guy solemnly answered, and that's where things got ugly.

Given the guy's black belt, he'd just committed aggravated assault. A kick to the head from a trained martial artist is reasonably likely to cause death or serious physical injury, so he was in just as much trouble as he would have been had he pulled a knife or a gun. Fortunately for everyone involved, the kick hadn't connected with its intended target. The fan, suddenly contrite, was given a choice: He could tell the officer who his *sifu* (instructor) was so that his unseemly behavior could be reported to his instructor, or he could be arrested for the assault. Interestingly enough, he selected jail as the safer choice. That says something about the character of his instructor.

Let's face it, high kicks look really cool. That's why they are often seen in tournament competitions and movie choreography. Unfortunately, these techniques are simply not practical in most real-world self-defense situations. Unless you are vastly more skilled or a lot faster than your adversary is, high kicks are not going to work.

When was the last time you had time to stretch out before a real fight? We certainly never have. No matter how flexible you are, it is fairly difficult to execute a high kick at full speed and power with cold muscles. Further, you are not necessarily going to be wearing loose-fitting clothing such as a karate *gi* the next time you find yourself in a real-world life-or-death encounter. The street clothes that most people wear are simply not conducive to the extreme leg movements necessary to kick above someone's waist. There's a reason competitors don't wear jeans in karate tournaments.

In the real world, self-defense entanglements typically happen fast, furiously, and at very close range. Balance and unimpaired movement are paramount when you tie up with an opponent. If you are knocked to the ground, you could easily be injured from the fall. Further, you can get stomped, maimed, or squashed like a bug while lying there momentarily defenseless.

Whenever you raise your foot high into the air, you take time to strike your opponent, weaken your balance, and very likely open yourself to counterattack. Low kicks to areas such as the feet, ankles, or knees, on the other hand, are much more effective due to the pain they inflict. They are harder to see and avoid, hence more likely to connect. Further, they do not disrupt your balance very much and can easily be performed in most regular street clothing.

From very close range, you can often strike with your knee, as *muay Thai* practitioners like to do, yet most of the time there's not even room for a full-on leg strike or kick. If you land a good shot from your knee and your opponent bends over from the impact, you can easily follow through with a kick from the foot, but still you never want to open with a high kick.

Once you have entangled an opponent's feet with your low kicks, you will have a much better chance of landing upper-body blows with your hand strikes. If you really want to kick him in the head, wait until you've knocked him to the ground first, and then do it. Watch your back legally, though; such actions might have adverse repercussions.

By the way, never try to kick a weapon. That's another thing that looks great in the movies but that can cost you dearly in the real world. For example, if he's got a knife, it takes only a quick flick of the wrist and you impale yourself on his blade. Unless you're some kind of superevolved mutant life-form, his hands are faster than your feet.

Don't Play "Tank"

Sadly, inexperienced fighters tend to stand in place while whaling away at each other without paying attention to evasive movement, stances, or mobility. You're not a heavily armored tank. It hurts to get hit. Consequently, standing toe-to-toe and duking it out with your adversary is just plain dumb, particularly if he's big, highly skilled, or armed.

The only time Kane has ever been sucker punched was at a college fraternity party in 1985. The guy who hit him was a twenty-two-year-old, 310-pound Samoan football player, a guy twice his weight and strong as an ox. Although the football player's blow caught him along the side of his jaw, knocking him to the ground, he was back on his feet doing his best Bruce Lee imitation seconds later.

The two flailed at each other for what seemed like several min-

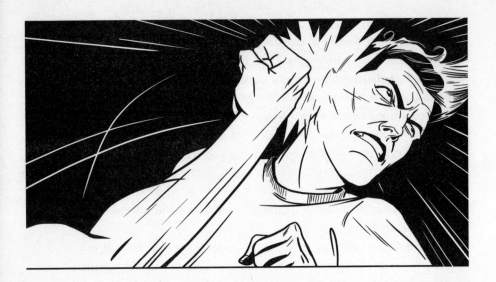

utes, trading blows, though it was probably much shorter than it seemed. While neither combatant realized it at that time, despite the Samoan's strength and Kane's agility, neither of them could throw a decent punch. They didn't move too well either. While Kane ultimately lost, he received only a sore jaw and a bloody nose. His opponent, who barely flinched under his best shot, wasn't injured either.

In retrospect, the thought of the two of them thumping on each other to no effect is pretty funny. By the time it was over, they held a grudging respect for each other's ability to take a punch and even became something like friends later on, yet not all fistfights end so sociably.

If you don't want to get hurt, you will need to move away from the strength of the other guy's attack. It is imperative to not only get off-line but also keep your attacker from being able to reorient immediately. Imagine someone holding a fist out like they just threw a punch. Now instead of standing directly in front of the blow, move diagonally toward the bad guy and to the side so that he will miss. Next, in addition to moving, shove his arm across his body so that it's no longer a threat. Martial artists call this "closing."

Closing is done by moving to the outside while blocking across the opponent's body to tie up his limbs, forcing him to reposition before counterattacking. Fighting "down the centerline" (the middle of the body) is very difficult to perfect, whereas moving offline and closing is taught to beginners because it is easier to learn. And it works pretty well too. It is even better if you can manage to get behind the other guy.

Use movement and distraction to unbalance and overcome. Stay balanced, upright, and mobile, keeping your weight centered over your feet. Body positioning and mobility not only keep you out of harm's way but also afford opportunities to counterstrike. Good balance is also needed if you are to generate powerful, effective techniques.

Don't let yourself get boxed in. Use mobility to control the distance and the angles between yourself and the other guy. While this is paramount for armed assaults, it is important for unarmed ones too. You're not a tank, so don't fight like one.

Don't Hit with a Closed Fist . . . Unless You've Got Skills

Unless you are an experienced martial artist, don't punch using a closed fist. The odds are good that you'll damage yourself at least as much as you will hurt your adversary. Even Mike Tyson, a guy who clearly knows how to hit, broke his hand in a street brawl when he hit fellow boxer Mitch Green incorrectly.* Furthermore, striking with a closed fist looks bad to potential witnesses, as it is an offensive technique.

Go ahead and test it for yourself. Find a brick or cement wall, make a good fist, and give it a light tap with your knuckles. Then slap it good and hard with your open hand. Which one hurts more?

If you insist on hitting with a closed fist, avoid targeting the other guy's face. Body shots are much less likely to damage your

---

* The incident took place in Harlem during August 1988.

hand, though you can still mess up your wrists if you hit incorrectly. Incidentally, that's why boxers tape their hands and wrists.

This brings us to the concept of contouring, an important component of street fighting that is commonly overlooked in martial arts training since it becomes irrelevant when safety gear and heavy gloves dramatically change the dynamics. Contouring helps you identify the best target for a given technique and can be summed up this way: Hard parts strike soft targets and soft parts strike hard targets.

Here's how it works: If you have ever punched someone in the jaw with your closed fist, you undoubtedly know how painful that can be for both parties. Hard fist to hard jaw is simply no good. We have seen quite a few broken knuckles resulting from such mistakes. A palm-heel strike to the jaw, on the other hand, can be quite effective. Soft palm to hard jaw is a good equation.

If you take a close look at all of your striking surfaces—your feet, hands, knees, and elbows—you can see how targeting works at a more granular level. For example, the blade edge (outside) of your foot aligns best with the other guy's joints (for example, the knee), while the ball of your foot makes a good fit with his groin or midsection, particularly if you use an upward arc when you strike. Different types of kicks are best for different targets.

The same thing applies to punches too. A single knuckle or finger strike fits the solar plexus better than the whole fist; the solar plexus is small, so by hitting with one or two fingers, the blow is concentrated into that area rather than dispersed as it would be with a fist. A hammer fist aligns much better with the temple or the forehead than it does with the base of the jaw or stomach, where an uppercut or palm-up straight punch might better apply.

Don't Forget to Use Your Mouth Too

If you have ever watched college or professional sports, you have no doubt seen instances in which one player fouls another, who subsequently retaliates. In the majority of those cases, it is the second player whom the referee observes committing the infraction. His eye is drawn toward the initial motion, yet he only notices the retaliatory strike. Consequently, the guy who started the confrontation gets off.

It works that way on the street as well. Witnesses frequently see the reaction of the victim and think that his defense is the first blow. Consequently, the person who initiates a fight is perceived as the good guy. This could be highly problematic when the police arrive or things get to court.

Look at how many police brutality cases there have been in recent years. Law enforcement officers are highly trained, following specific policies and procedures, yet they are frequently accused of overreacting. How much more likely is the average civilian, who has no policy or procedure to follow, to be similarly accused of wrongdoing?

If you want to protect yourself, you need to make sure that everyone around you knows that you are the good guy in the fight. So how can you create a witness who is likely to interpret your just actions favorably? You create witnesses by using your mouth as a weapon. It can be just as potent as your fists or feet in a fight and often proves more important in the long run.

Start by acting afraid—you probably are anyway—by verbally calling for help. There is an off chance that you can ward off your assailant or convince someone to intervene on your behalf simply by shouting for help. Even if you can't, you might still convince others around that you are the good guy. Shouting something along the lines of, "Oh my God, don't kill me with that knife!" is a pretty good indicator of peril. It clearly differentiates you from the other guy and should help justify your use of force in court if it gets that far.

"I don't want to fight you," "Please don't hurt me," "Put down the weapon," and "Help, he's got a gun" all put you in a much better light than "Go ahead, make my day!" or "I'm gonna kill you, sucker!" Think about various scenarios ahead of time so that you will have a better chance of articulating strategically. It is pretty easy to shout something during a fight. The real challenge is finding words that put you in the best possible light and your assailant in the worst. In other words, it is easy to shout but hard to verbalize strategically, so you need to practice this. Many martial arts classes do role-playing and scenario drills that give you the opportunity to exercise your verbal skills while fighting.

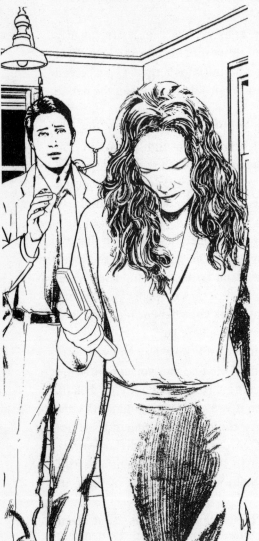

What you say before, during, and after a confrontation is important. If, for example, you knock your attacker to the ground, then proceed to kick or pummel him, you will be seen as overreacting, even in many cases where you are on sound tactical ground. A far better tactic would be to precede any further action with verbal commands such as "Stay down," "Stop fighting me," or "Drop the weapon."

Your mouth is an important weapon. Don't forget to use it.

Don't Play the Other Guy's Game

Darrell, a burly 200-pound logger friend of Wilder's, had a very near miss. His chain saw tangled on a log, bucked up, and bounced toward his throat. The good news is that he saved his life by blocking the running saw blade with his hand. The bad news is that he blocked a running saw blade with his hand. His palm was torn up pretty good.

A week or so later, before the injury had healed very much, he decided to go drinking with some friends, trying to unwind. Unfortunately, he ran afoul of another guy who was spoiling for a fight. The bully saw Darrell's injury and hoped to take advantage of his weakness. This other guy was big, maybe even a bit bigger than Darrell, yet he wasn't used to getting up at the crack of dawn, climbing up and down hills through the woods, and wrestling logs for a living. He came on strong, but the fight was short. Using his left, uninjured hand, Darrell picked the other guy up, carried him flailing in the air for half a dozen steps, and tossed him out the door down a flight of stairs.

As the bully found out, it doesn't pay to play the other guy's game. The bully was used to being the stronger guy, but he ran across a guy who was not only stronger but sore, tired, and irritable as well. When you're going to fight a big guy, it doesn't make sense to face him toe-to-toe.

No matter how big you are, there's always somebody bigger. No matter how strong, there's always somebody stronger. If you're used to playing the big-guy game of simply overpowering someone and that's all you've got, you're in for a nasty surprise when you find yourself the smaller or weaker man. If you're going to train to fight, you need to understand both the big guy's and the little guy's role. There are different strategies for each, and knowing how to fight in either role is key. While you cannot fight him down the middle if you're overmatched, you can still break him down from the outside. If he's big, fight like a small guy, and vice versa.

The size differential is but one aspect of disparity in a fight. The other has to do with your training and natural tendencies.

Here's how it works: Let's say for the sake of argument that you're a striker. Maybe you study boxing or karate. While the art of karate encompasses grappling, throwing, pressure points, and submission applications, it's primarily a striking style, attacking with fists, elbows, and open-hand techniques. If that's your strength, use it. Get close, throw a lot of punches and maybe a short kick or two, and pound the other guy into submission so that you can escape to safety.

Tae kwon do practitioners, on the other hand, are very good with their feet. If you're a hand striker, tangling up in kicking range would be a recipe for disaster. That's playing to the other guy's strength. You'd need to get in close to take away his range advantage in order to do the most damage with your hand techniques. Similarly, judoka and jujitsu practitioners will want to go "ground and pound," knocking you down and busting up your joints or choking you into submission. That's their game, not yours. It's very hard to throw an effective punch when you're lying flat on your back with the wind knocked out of you. Watch just about any Mixed Martial Arts (MMA) match and you'll see good examples of that.

It's foolhardy to think that you can overcome an adversary by using the style he's better at. Play your game, not the other guy's.

Don't Use the Wrong Technique for the Situation

When Kane first began training in karate, he was frequently matched up with another practitioner named Mike. Working toward their green belt tests, they repeatedly performed a prearranged tandem sparring drill using techniques from one of the kata (forms) that they were supposed to know on the test. One of these sequences called for a front kick toward the groin from one partner, while the other guy turned his body to pull his family jewels off the line of attack while simultaneously sweeping aside and deflecting the kick with his arm.

Kane and Mike worked this drill during and after class for several weeks, reaching a point where they could perform it swiftly and well, or so they thought. One day they had the opportunity to perform this drill with Scott, a visiting black belt. Kane went first. When Scott threw the front kick, Kane took a solid strike to the groin. He realized that during their friendly practice sessions, he and Mike had subconsciously aimed their kicks away from each other, eliminating the need to seriously block the techniques. Turning their bodies a little was all it took to avoid getting hit by these unaimed strikes. Since the deflections were relatively unnecessary, they had not been training realistically even though they thought they had been. The first properly aimed, full-speed blow painfully pointed out that shortcoming. Thankfully, it happened on the practice floor rather than in combat on the street.

If you expect to do well in a fight, you must examine what you are doing through the lens of an opponent rather than a training partner. The other guy is going to be doing his damnedest to sabotage whatever it is that you want to do. And he wants to hurt you in the process.

Notice that these are all striking techniques, the kind of stuff that boxers, tae kwon do practitioners, and *karateka* like to employ. Hitting someone in a street fight is a good way to retain your mobility. When you are moving and striking, you are much safer than when you're slugging it out in place or rolling around grappling. Although many locks and holds can be applied standing up if you have sufficient training, the majority are most effective when applied to an adversary on the ground. It is simply easier to control the guy's movement or immobilize him that way. The problem is that if you go to the ground in a self-defense situation and your opponent has any friends around, you have put yourself in an extremely vulnerable position.

This means that locks, holds, and throws have limited utility in most street fights. They can certainly be used in the right situations, but by no means universally. Be very sure that the tactical situation warrants such applications before attempting them outside the tournament hall. It's not just going to the ground or constricting your ability to move and escape that you need to worry about.

Adrenaline robs you of fine motor coordination in a fight, so you have to keep things simple and direct. Finger locks, for example, are great parlor tricks. They're eminently painful, and you can latch on to a victim and really make him dance with one, yet they are virtually impossible to pull off in a real fight, particularly when sweat, blood, pepper spray, or other slippery substances are thrown into the mix. While precise grabbing movements are extraordinarily tough, even imprecise ones like grabbing a wrist or hooking a leg can be problematic unless you're highly trained. If you try to get too fancy or precise, you will dramatically hurt your chances for success.

However, gross motor movements, especially those that target vital areas of the adversary's body, work pretty well. Applications on the street just don't work the same as they do in the training hall, in part because you are fighting an adversary who's doing his all-out best to defeat you. It's tough enough to get in a few solid blows without getting thumped yourself; don't compound the mistake by trying the wrong thing.

Don't Go to the Ground

Avoid going to the ground in a fight. The ground is where you can easily get stomped, kicked, and maimed, if not killed. If you land on the ground, get up as fast as you can. Grapplers will tell you

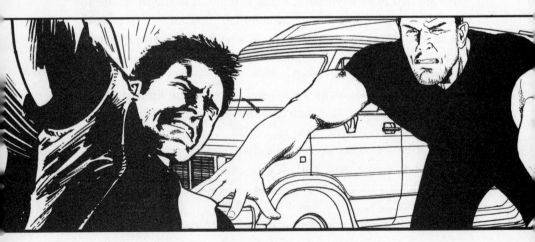

that submission techniques, or "ground and pound," are great means to end a fight. They are absolutely correct . . . in the tournament ring. On the street they are flat-out wrong.

Going to the ground in a real fight puts you in a position where your adversary can easily stomp a mud hole in you. Even if he chooses not to do so or drops down with you to grapple, his buddies will most likely put the boots to you. Or his girlfriend will. Either way, you are in dire straits; the ground is a very bad place to be.

Sitting in a bar one day, Wilder watched a conversation between two men at an adjoining table grow in intensity. As they argued, these men sat side by side, turned slightly toward each other. One of them was wearing a white T-shirt. Without any telegraphing of his intentions, White T-shirt Guy suddenly reached up behind the other man's head and grabbed a wad of hair. Grip secured, he stood up and jerked the other guy down to the floor.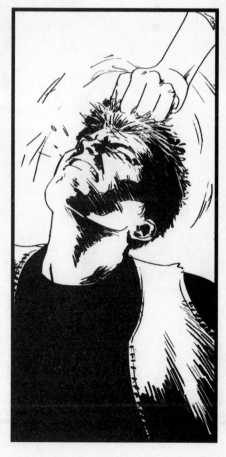

In the one deft motion, he put the other guy down hard. Mr. T-shirt spread both hands out, supporting his weight between two tables, and swiftly kicked the other guy six or seven times in the face. Before anyone could react, he launched himself forward and ran from the bar.

The elapsed time for the entire fight was, perhaps, four or five seconds. By the time it was over, the other guy needed serious dental work and a few dozen stitches. This is a good example of how being on the ground will get you stomped.

And if you think you want to be doing the stomping, like White T-shirt Guy, listen up. One of our students came into the dojo one night and told us the story of a fight at his high school. When one student hit the ground, the other guy managed to remain standing. He used this advantage to kick his fallen opponent viciously several times in the head hard enough to dislocate the other kid's eye. His kicks crushed the bone in the side of the other kid's head, collapsed the eye socket, and popped out the eyeball.

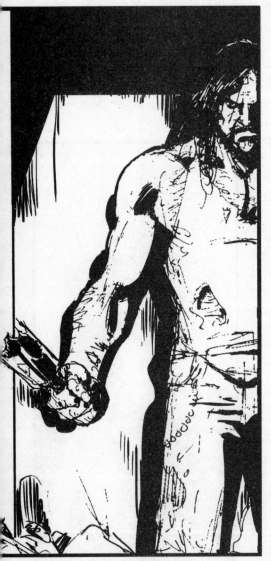

The kid who did the kicking, oh, he had been in trouble before, in and out of juvenile detention several times in his young life. This particular fight happened just after his eighteenth birthday, however, so his reality shifted a bit. Suddenly he faced aggravated assault charges, cooling his heels with other incarcerated adults until his trial. He enjoyed Thanksgiving, Christmas, and New Year's in jail. He not only missed his high school graduation but also faced a five-to-seven-year prison term.

Try to get a decent job with no high school diploma or to rent an apartment after you have checked the *yes* box, which is on every apartment rental application, where it asks, "Have you ever been convicted of a felony?"

Ever seen the victim of a Berkeley stomp? That's when a guy is shoved up against a curb with his mouth wrapped around the cement. He is then kicked in the back of the head, fracturing the jaw and knocking out his teeth.

It's ugly. Perhaps not quite as bad as having your eyeball popped out from the force of a blow, but ugly enough.

The ground you fight on may be unsafe too. For example, an alley strewn with garbage, broken glass, used condoms, and discarded syringes is a breeding ground for all kinds of nasty diseases, many of which can be transmitted through open wounds. Falling on concrete, rocks, broken branches, or sharp debris can cause serious injuries. And your adversary may grab something lying on the ground and use it as an impromptu weapon, taking the fight to a whole new level.

The only people who can safely go to the ground in a real fight are police officers, security personnel, and other people who work in highly trained, well-coordinated teams. As one or more officers take down, control, and restrain the subject, the rest secure the perimeter so that they will not be overly vulnerable during the process. Unless you are a skilled professional working with an experienced team, the ground is a dangerous place to be.

CHAPTER ELEVEN

Things to Keep in Mind

Never Hit a Girl . . . Unless She's Armed

While experienced bouncers, bodyguards, law enforcement officers, soldiers, jail guards, and martial artists know that women can
be just as dangerous, or possibly even more so, as men,* the courts
don't often see it that way. If the "big, burly man" strikes the "tiny,
helpless woman," even in a case of legitimate self-defense, judges
and juries will naturally see the size, gender, and strength differential and take that into account. Stuff like that usually ends badly.

Gender differences can become particularly challenging if
you are caught by surprise. Because of your "fight-or-flight" reflex,
it can be normal to lash out responsively. If you have an occupation
that deals with violence on a regular basis, you may be somewhat
better prepared from long experience. Regardless, excess caution
in such instances is almost always prudent. Act as if you are on live
television. Who knows, with all the camera phones, video cameras,

---

* Such as instinctively going for the eyes during an attack.

closed-circuit televisions, and recording technology out there, perhaps you are on tape.

The cornerstone of a legitimate claim of self-defense is the innocence of the claimant. You must be entirely without fault. If you initiate the conflict, you cannot claim self-defense. If you allow a conflict to escalate into a lethal situation when it could have been avoided, you share some degree of culpability and, once again, cannot claim self-defense.

Depending on the circumstances, almost any form of physical assault can be considered deadly force. In Washington State, deadly force is defined as "the intentional application of force through the use of firearms or any other means reasonably likely to cause death or serious physical injury."* Other jurisdictions will have similar definitions. In general, any blow delivered powerfully and deliberately to a vital part of the body may be construed as deadly force so long as it can be shown that it was struck with the intention, or predictable likelihood, of killing. That means that simply smacking someone upside the head could conceivably be considered deadly force.

The courts are more likely to interpret a blow as deadly force if the person delivering it is physically much stronger than the victim. If you're a professional fighter, a trained martial artist, or attacking with extreme savagery,† you're going to have a tough time claiming self-defense. Unfortunately, that "physically stronger than the victim" part is rather hard to avoid if you are a male fighting a female, unless you are fairly small or she is unusually large.

Equal force doctrines require a law-abiding citizen to respond to an attack with little force or no more than that which he perceives is being used against him. In some places, the law clearly specifies that equal force must be exactly equal. The attacked can respond with no more force than that by which he

---

* Revised Code of Washington, RCW 9A.16.010.

† An example of "extreme savagery" in the eyes of the law would be gratuitously raining blows upon a fallen opponent who has obviously given up the conflict, even if he started the fight in the first place.

is threatened—slap for slap, punch for punch, kick for kick, or deadly weapon for deadly weapon. Once again, that's pretty tough if you're a guy and your adversary is a girl. Whatever you do may easily be perceived as figurative or literal overkill. Everything changes when weapons are involved, however. An armed opponent clearly has the advantage, so you have much more leeway in your response.

Disparity of force between unarmed combatants is measured in one of two ways. It exists if (1) the victim is being attacked by someone who is physically much stronger or younger, or (2) the victim is being attacked by two or more assailants of similar or equal size. In such cases, you may legitimately be able to exert potentially lethal force to defend yourself. Regardless, nowhere can a person legally respond to an assault of slight degree with deadly force.

A great majority of states require that law-abiding citizens avoid conflict whenever possible. It is best to withdraw, leaving the scene entirely. It is always a good idea to retreat from a belligerent party who threatens you, unless the attack is so savage that there is not sufficient time to escape or unless withdrawing (or leaving cover in the case of a gunfight) would increase your vulnerability.

The only exception to this rule is within the confines of your own home (or in some jurisdictions your place of business). In most cases, if someone breaks into your home and assaults you, you do not legally need to attempt to retreat. In many cases, it may be prudent to do so anyway, however. This is not true in all jurisdictions, though, so check your local laws carefully. This statute is often called a "castle doctrine."

The bottom line is that in the eyes of the court, you must be in reasonable fear for your life or someone else's prior to applying countervailing force. That's awful hard to prove if the other guy is a girl, unless she's armed with some sort of weapon. If you are cornered and have to fight, you clearly do whatever you have to in order to assure your safety and well-being. It is essential, however, to make a commitment to yourself to use physical force wisely. Never hit a girl . . . unless she's armed.

As Stress Goes Up, Intelligence Goes Down

When adrenaline hits your system, you become tougher and more resilient, but the downside is that you become a one-task, knuckle-dragging troglodyte. Your ability to think rationally is reduced, you lose your peripheral vision, and your hearing is impaired.

The New York Police Department did a comprehensive analysis of police-involved shooting incidents, evaluating some six thousand violent altercations that took place during the 1970s. Ninety percent of those shootings took place at distances of less than fifteen feet. They found that officers hit their targets roughly a quarter of the time, while criminal assailants made about 11 percent of their shots. Highly trained professionals who near universally hit their targets in practice missed 75 percent of their shots during live fire situations. Criminals who presumably had less experience handling firearms missed 89 percent of the time.

Not all hits were fatal. During the period of 1970 through 1979, law enforcement officers inflicted ten casualties for every one suffered at the hands of their criminal assailants. In all of the cases investigated, the size, shape, configuration, composition, caliber, and velocity of the bullet was not the preeminent factor in determining who lived or died. Shot placement was the overarching cause of death,* which is clear evidence that adrenal stress must be overcome to survive a street fight.

The more stressed you are through exertion, fear, or desperation, the harder it is to perform. In a violent encounter, your heart rate can jump from 60 or 70 beats per minute (BPM) to well over 200 BMP in less than half a second. Here is how accelerated heart rates can affect you:

■ For people whose resting heart rate is around 60 to 70 BPM, at around 115 BPM many begin to lose fine motor skills such as finger dexterity, making it difficult to successfully dial a phone, open a lock, or aim a weapon.

---

* Or injuries serious enough to end the confrontation.

■ Around 145 BPM, most people begin to lose their complex motor skills such as hand-eye coordination, precise tracking movements, or exact timing, making complicated techniques very challenging if not impossible.

■ Around 175 BPM, most people begin to lose depth perception, experience tunnel vision, and sometimes even suffer temporary memory loss.

■ Around 185–220 BPM, many people experience hypervigilance, loss of rational thought, and inability to consciously move or react. Without prior training, the vast majority of people cannot function at this stress level.

Breath control techniques can help you recover from the effects of adrenaline to a large degree, though it takes much practice to control your breathing in a fight. Here's how it works: Breathe in through your nose, let the air swirl around in your belly, and then breathe out through your mouth. Break the breath into three components, clearly inhaling, holding, and exhaling with a four-count pause in between each step. In other words, each cycle of combat breathing includes:

- *Inhale for a four-count.*
- *Hold for a four-count.*
- *Exhale for a four-count.*

This process helps you oxygenate your blood while psychologically calming you during extreme stress. Nevertheless, it's important not to take unnecessary risks. Since it's tough to focus on more than one thing, escape should be your primary goal. As stress goes up, intelligence goes down.

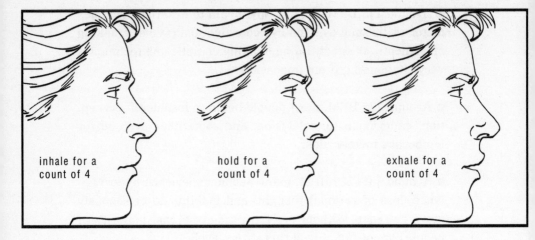

inhale for a
count of 4

hold for a
count of 4

exhale for a
count of 4

When He Stops, You Stop

There is a hilarious scene in the movie *Monty Python and the Holy Grail* where the legendary King Arthur battles the dreaded Black Knight. Wielding Excalibur, Arthur is an invincible warrior, easily cleaving off his adversary's arm. Thinking the battle has been won, Arthur begins to celebrate his victory, yet the Black Knight responds, "'Tis but a flesh wound," and continues to battle. This continues until Arthur has hacked off both of the Black Knight's arms as well as his legs and subsequently begins to ride away, leaving his defenseless adversary behind. Unwilling to yield, however, the Black Knight screams, "Come back! I'll bite your knees off!" Clearly, this is a comedic fantasy, yet it has some bearing in real life.

If someone's heart is truly in a fight, strikes to his nonvital areas can have very little effect. It is extremely tough to stop a determined foe. Loren Christensen wrote, "I've had to fight guys even after they have been shot and they still fought like maniacs. I know of two occasions where suspects had been shot in their hearts and they fought the officers for several seconds before they crumpled dead to the ground. . . . I saw two cases of people shot in the head—one person took five rounds—and they were still running around screaming and putting up a fuss."

Unless you are a master martial artist who can deliver hydrostatic shock that disrupts internal organs with each blow—something that takes a good ten to twenty years of dedicated training to learn, let alone perfect—it is really hard to beat somebody down without resorting to a weapon. Either you need to shock the brain stem into shutting down with a knockout blow or you need to break darn near every bone in his body, delivering such extensive physiological damage that it is physically impossible for him to continue fighting. The vast majority of opponents, however, will give up long before you get to that point. Once they stop, you need to stop too. Remain wary in case the other guy changes his mind, of course, but break off your attack and move to a safer location.

One master of strategy, Sun Tzu, tells you to leave a way out for your enemy, saying, "When you surround an army, leave an outlet free. Do not press a desperate foe too hard." This is sound advice because most people who find themselves with their back to the wall, faced with no options but to die or die fighting, will choose to fight and fight hard. You really don't want to mess with a fully committed foe.

Here is the way it breaks down. If a punk decides to fight with you, whatever the reason, you have a right to defend yourself—to a point. If you beat the punk down so that he has stopped fighting with you, you have to stop as well. The classic rule is that self-defense begins when deadly danger begins, ends when the danger ends, and revives again if the danger returns. Neither a killing nor a beating that takes place after a crime has already been committed, nor a proactive violent defense before an attack has taken place, is legitimately self-defense in the eyes of the law.

You can only resort to deadly or potentially deadly force to escape imminent and unavoidable danger of death or grave bodily harm. An attacker must not merely have made a threat to attack you but must also be in a position where he or she is obviously and immediately capable of carrying out that threat and/or has begun to do so. A common test is that the attacker must demonstrate intent to attack and have both the means and opportunity to do so. Once he breaks off his assault, you must stop yours too.

When You Stop, He Won't Stop

When you stop, there is no guarantee that the other guy will too. You are taking a monumental risk if you roll up into a ball on the ground and assume that your submission will end the fight. This may be taken as nothing more than a green light for the other guy to stomp you . . . a lot. In fact, you can pretty much count on it.

The only way you can stop a fight when you are losing is to escape. Run away as fast and as far as you can. Do not stop; do not look behind you, at least not right away; just run. It is really tough to capture someone who is bound and determined to get away. It's not just a factor of speed but also of terror. When the shooting starts, you'd be amazed by how fast you can move. The same thing holds true for a fistfight; use this to your advantage.

Breaking off your attack, in and of itself, is probably not going to end the fight, particularly if the other guy wants to be in control. His goal is complete and utter dominance over you, supremacy for all to see. You cannot count on honor, ethics, or mercy from an adversary. If you depend on his good nature, you are bound to lose the fight in a very bad way. It is smart to show honor yourself yet prudent to expect none from your opponent.

The best way to avoid getting beaten down is not to fight in the first place. If you cannot escape violence, however, you must fight with all you're worth. Your goal does not necessarily need to be to win, but it must at least be to not lose. In other words, you don't need to beat the other guy to a pulp, but you do need to escape successfully. That is not going to happen if you give up the struggle. If you stop, there's no guarantee that he will too.

SECTION THREE

AFTERMATH OF VIOLENCE

Man is Buddha—
the day and I
grow dark as one.
—RYUSHI (1684-1764)[4]

This section covers the aftermath of violence, showing that it's almost never over when it's over. We're going to assume, for the sake of argument, that once the dust has settled, you are still alive. Otherwise, there won't be much aftermath for you to deal with; that'll be left for the authorities and your mourners to hash out.

The bad news is that living through the fight is just the beginning. There are a host of other consequences to address, including first aid, legal issues, managing witnesses, finding a good attorney, dealing with the press, interacting with law enforcement, and dealing with psychological trauma.

If you were unexpectedly attacked, were ambushed with a weapon, or suddenly discovered that what you thought would be a simple fistfight had escalated into something far more serious, you will need to get your head in the right place after it's over. You may be gravely wounded and/or facing serious short- and long-term repercussions. Your first order of business must be to know your priorities and act accordingly.

CHAPTER TWELVE

Once It's Over, Know Your Priorities

Once you survive a violent conflict, your first order of business must be your continued survival. If you have been injured during a fight, you may have to take care of yourself until professional help can arrive. First, you need to make a mental commitment to live. Your attitude plays a large part in your ability to survive. It's also important to know how to treat your own injuries, as you may be on your own for a long time until paramedics or other assistance arrive.

Once you have taken care of any life-threatening injuries, you will want to turn your attention to notifying the authorities; calling your attorney; contacting your wife, girlfriend, or appropriate family member; and identifying any witnesses who may be able to testify about your actions and those of your adversary.

While you may or may not have to fight to work through and recover from injuries and/or emotional scars, you almost certainly will have to fight for your freedom and livelihood in court. Your defense begins before the altercation gets physical and often doesn't end for months or years to come. While the opening salvo is playing to any witnesses who might see the fight or to video equipment that might record what happens, one of the most important skirmishes will be your first contact with the police.

When the authorities arrive, approach the responding officers calmly and politely. A confrontational attitude will do you no good. Follow the officers' instructions without hesitation. Expect to be arrested. It may or may not happen, but if you are arrested, do not resist for any reason. Similarly, do not interfere with an attempt to arrest anyone who is with you at the time.

Do not, under any circumstances, make any incriminating statements that may be used against you at a later time. Despite Miranda[5] requirements, your fundamental rights and responsibilities may not always be clearly spelled out by the responding officers, especially in any conversations that precede an arrest. Your priority should be to alleviate or minimize any potential charges against you, so be enormously cautious about what you say and do.

The legal process is arduous, complicated, and expensive. It generally begins with an arrest followed by a booking, arraignment, evidentiary hearing, and trial. At times, an appeal will be necessary as well. Because your freedom, family, livelihood, and reputation are on the line, it is essential to have a highly skilled and experienced attorney to help you navigate the process. You should always carry the phone number of an attorney you can trust and of a person who can contact a lawyer for you if yours is not immediately available. That means, of course, that you will need to be proactive and find an attorney before you need one.

Killing or crippling another human being is traumatic, even when it's absolutely the right thing to do in order to preserve your own life and well-being. The other guy might be a total scumbag while he's attacking you, but he's still a person, someone with a family, friends, and loved ones who will miss him when he's gone. For example, serial killer Ted Bundy's mother's last words to him were, "You will always be my precious son." She said that right before he was executed by the State of Florida for his crimes.*

---

* Theodore Robert Bundy (1946-1989) was one of the most infamous serial killers in U.S. history. While Bundy confessed to raping and murdering some

If you put someone down on the street, there is no legal process, proceeding, or appeal. There is no judge or jury, only an executioner. You fight. You win. He dies. Sure, lesser outcomes are certainly possible, but it's important to prepare yourself mentally for that ultimate eventuality. It all takes place in the blink of an eye, yet you'll remember it for the rest of your life if it goes that far. Win or lose, there's always a cost to engaging in violence.

---

thirty women before his execution, his total number of victims remains unknown.

CHAPTER THIRTEEN

Know How to Perform First Aid

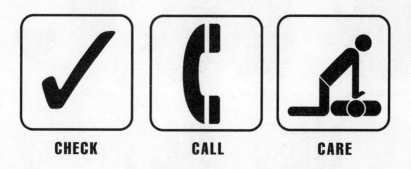

CHECK   CALL   CARE

Even if you don't expect to get into a fight, it's a good idea to know what to do if you or a loved one becomes injured. The Red Cross and Red Crescent provide relatively inexpensive, comprehensive first-aid and CPR classes throughout the world, so access to training is rarely a problem. It is also important to keep emergency supplies in your home and carry a first-aid kit in your vehicle. It's pretty tough to patch yourself up if you don't have the proper equipment available. Be sure to include rubber gloves to protect yourself from blood-borne pathogens (e.g., hepatitis B, hepatitis C, or HIV/AIDS) if you have to treat others as well.

Once you have taken care of your own life-threatening injuries, you will also want to treat your opponent. Remember that your goal in applying countervailing force is to keep yourself safe from harm. If your adversary is disabled and no longer a threat, it is both prudent and humane to try to keep him from dying from his wounds. It may play well in court too.

There are far too many wounds that victims might receive to cover them all, but we've included details about how to deal with some of the most common ones below. This information is only an introduction and should never take the place of professional, hands-on instruction.

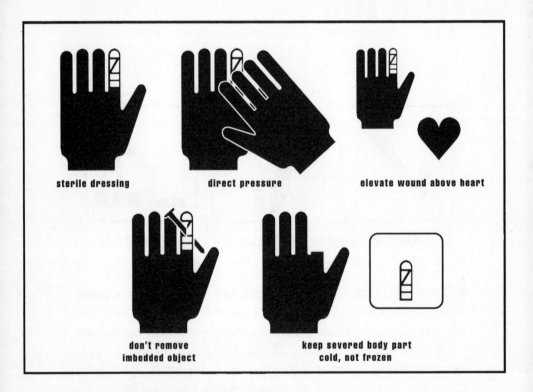

sterile dressing

direct pressure

elevate wound above heart

don't remove
imbedded object

keep severed body part
cold, not frozen

Control Bleeding

Heavy bleeding is often the most serious, life-threatening injury victims can receive in a fight. One of the most street-proven trauma dressings is a sanitary napkin or a box of Kleenex, something that ought to be in your first-aid kit in addition to regular gauze pads and bandages. Key first-aid methods for stopping heavy bleeding include:

■ Covering the wound with a sterile dressing such as a gauze pad. If the dressing becomes soaked with blood, apply additional layers over the top of it without removing the original dressing.

■ Applying direct pressure to the wound. If bleeding does not stop through a combination of dressings and pressure, remove the dressings, pack the wound with QuikClot (or a similar hemostatic agent), and reapply new sterile dressings. Use a pressure bandage to hold everything in place if available. If you do not have access to specialty agents, you may have to apply direct pressure to a nearby artery to slow the flow of blood. On the arm, the best point is along the inside of the upper arm between the shoulder and elbow. On the leg, the best point is at the crease at the front of the hip in the groin area.

■ Elevating the wound above the level of the heart if possible. If you suspect head, neck, or back injuries or broken bones, however, it may be prudent to remain in place. Moving may increase the severity of the damage.

■ Never removing embedded objects before you get to the hospital. Doing so may increase hemorrhaging and severely reduce your chances of survival. Bulky dressings should be placed around the object and bandaged in place to support it so that it won't move around and cause further damage.

■ Wrapping severed body parts, if any, in a sterile dressing, placing them in a plastic bag, and covering them with ice or cold water sufficient to keep the parts cool without freezing. Limbs preserved in this manner can frequently be reattached at the hospital. On the other hand, freezing the severed part will cause irreversible damage.

Head, Neck, and Back Injuries

Head, neck, and back injuries are serious. Do not move the victim unless necessary. If you do need to move the person, be careful to support the injured area, avoiding any twisting, bending, or other contortions that could cause additional damage. If the person becomes unconscious, you will need to maintain a clear airway and possibly perform rescue breathing or cardiopulmonary resuscitation.

Concussions

The brain is delicate yet protected by a rigid skull and cushioned with cerebrospinal fluid. Trauma to the head can cause the brain to bounce against the skull. This force may damage the brain's function. There is very little extra room within this cavity, so any resulting swelling or bleeding can quickly become life threatening. In general, a blow to the front of the head is less dangerous than one on the side or back of the head.

Symptoms of a concussion can include severe headache, dizziness, nausea, vomiting, ringing in the ears, mismatched pupil size (left versus right), seizures, or slurred speech. The person may also seem restless, agitated, or irritable. Often, the victim may experience temporary memory loss. These symptoms may last from hours to weeks, depending on the seriousness of the injury.

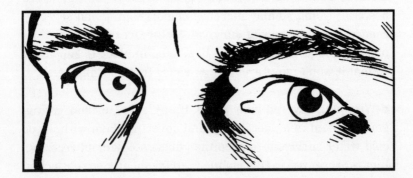

Watch the person closely for any changes in level of consciousness until medical help arrives. Anyone knocked out from a head injury must be evaluated by medical professionals. The victim may need to stay in the hospital for close observation. Although the symptoms tend to go away over time, some victims will need a rehabilitation specialist to oversee a program for their recovery.

People who have had a severe concussion also double their risk of developing epilepsy within the first five years after the injury. There is evidence that people who have had multiple concussions over the course of their lives suffer cumulative neurological damage. A link between concussions and the eventual development of Alzheimer's disease also has been suggested.

Rest is generally the best recovery technique, since healing a concussion takes time. For headaches, acetaminophen (Tylenol) or ibuprofen (Motrin) can usually be used, but it is best to avoid aspirin as it can increase the risk of internal bleeding. Check with a doctor before administering medications. Bumps and contusions can be treated with ice packs. Wrap ice in a damp cloth rather than placing it directly against the skin.

Eye Injuries

Do not attempt to treat severe blunt trauma or penetrating injuries to the eye yourself; medical assistance is required in such instances. Tape a paper or Styrofoam cup over the injured area to protect it until proper care can be obtained. If there is an embedded object, do not attempt to remove it.

In the case of a blow to the eye, such as a finger rake, jab, or gouge, do not assume that the injury is minor even if you can see properly afterward. An ophthalmologist should examine the eye because vision-threatening damage, for example a detached retina, could be hidden. Apply an ice compress or bag of frozen vegetables (e.g., peas) to the eye to reduce pain and swelling. If you experience pain, blurred vision, floaters (black spots that move around), starbursts (firework-like bursts of color or light), or any possibility of eye damage, see your ophthalmologist or emergency room physician immediately.

Chest Wounds

Large chest wounds can cause a lung to collapse, a dangerous situation. Cover the wound with a sterile dressing or clean cloth and bandage it in place. If bubbles begin forming around a wound of significant size (an open area that is greater than about an inch in diameter), cover that area with plastic or similar material that does not allow air to pass through. Tape the dressing in place, leaving one corner open to allow air to escape with exhalation.

Most normal stab and bullet injuries will not cause a sucking chest wound, because the hole from the wound is smaller than the opening in the trachea. Consequently, it will not cause negative pressure, which inhibits breathing. If you seal a wound that does not need it, you run the risk of tension pneumothorax, which can cause complete cardio-respiratory arrest and subsequent death. If advanced medical care is readily available, it is generally more important to transport the victim to the hospital quickly than it is to seal off the wound with anything more than a breathable sterile dressing.

Abdominal Injuries

For abdominal injuries, try to keep the victim lying down with his or her knees bent if possible. If organs are exposed, do not apply pressure to the organs or push them back inside. Remove any clothing from around the wound. Apply moist, sterile dressings or clean cloth loosely over the wound. Keep the dressing moist with clean, warm water. Place a cloth over the dressing to keep the organs warm.

Broken Bones

Broken bones should usually be splinted to keep the injured part from moving and increasing the damage. There is a variety of ways to create an effective splint. The method you choose will be based in part on what materials you have available, the position you find the injury, its location on the body, and a variety of other factors. The most important thing is to pad and immobilize the injury to the extent possible. A basic rule of splinting is that the joints above and below the broken bone should be immobilized to protect the fracture site. For example, if the lower leg is broken, the splint should immobilize both the ankle and the knee.

Anatomic splints affix the injured body part to a convenient uninjured one, such as tying one leg to the other. A soft splint can be made from a towel, blanket, jacket, or similar material. A rigid splint can be made from boards, tightly rolled magazines, and similar materials.

Shock

Shock can occur whenever there is severe injury to the body or the nervous system. Because shock can cause inadequate blood flow to the tissues and organs, all bodily processes can be affected. Vital functions slow down to dangerous levels. In the early stages, the body compensates for a decreased blood flow to the tissues by constricting blood vessels in the skin, soft tissues, and muscles. This causes the victim to have cold, clammy, or pale skin; weakness and nausea; rapid, labored breathing; an increased pulse rate; and decreased blood pressure. As shock progresses, the victim will become apathetic and relatively unresponsive, and will eventually lapse into unconsciousness.

One quick and dirty way to identify shock is by observing a delayed capillary refill response at the fingertips. Press downward on the tip of the fingernail until the skin underneath begins to turn white, and then release the pressure. A normal pink appearance should return within two to three seconds. If it takes four to six seconds or longer for normal color to return, the victim is experiencing low blood pressure at the extremities, a clear sign of shock.

You should have already treated any major injuries such as bleeding or broken bones before treating for shock. This care will help ameliorate the source of the shock, but there is more that you can do. Keep the victim lying down, elevate his legs about a foot or so above his chest, and cover him with a blanket or coat to prevent loss of body heat. If the femur (thighbone) has been broken from a gunshot or blunt trauma injury, however, do not elevate the injured leg, as bone fragments may shift around and cause serious internal bleeding. Check the victim's airway, breathing, and circulation on a regular basis until medical help arrives. It is not advisable to give liquids to shock victims.

Infection

If you have been injured by a weapon that breaks the skin, infection is a possibility even after medical treatment. If the wound area becomes red or swollen, throbs with pain, discharges pus, or develops red streaks, contact medical personnel immediately. If you begin to develop a fever, it may also be a sign of infection. Seek direction from your physician as to how to bandage your injury, how frequently to change the dressing, and how best to clean the wound to minimize the chances of infection.

It's smart to learn first aid. Even if you never have to use it to care for yourself, odds are good that you will find opportunities to help others. If you study martial arts and learn how to hurt other people, it's even more important to understand how to help them as well.

CHAPTER FOURTEEN

Don't Exaggerate, Don't Threaten

"They have never hung a mute. Anything you say can and will be used against you in a court of law." That is what an attorney told Wilder some fifteen years ago. He was right then and he is right now. Don't exaggerate; it will be interpreted in the worst light when it is read in court. And don't threaten, because there is no question, no doubt without exception, that it is going to be used against you in court. Celebrities, politicians, and other powerful individuals often attempt to throw their weight around when dealing with the police, thinking that their name, reputation, or wealth will buy them special treatment. Despite some notorious and highly publicized exceptions, it usually ends badly for them and almost certainly will for you too, if you try to go that route.

When the police arrive, they will talk to everybody and write down everything they hear. What is written is neither screened nor reviewed. It is put into the report and the report goes into the official record. Any half-truths, lies, or whatever you utter will get written down and will be read into court as fact. Don't hang yourself with your own words.

Officers are there to ascertain the truth, gathering unbiased facts and evidence about what transpired. They are not there to hand you a medal for heroism under adversity even if you acted heroically. If, in their best judgment, there is probable cause that you should be locked up because you committed a crime, then that's exactly what will happen. Not exactly fair, but common enough nevertheless.

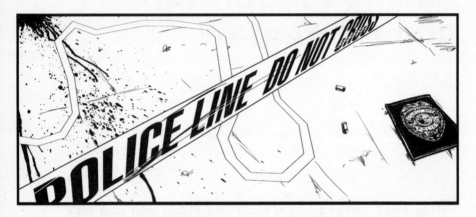

Approach the responding officer(s) positively. Police are people too. They likely have the same emotional makeup that you do. Officers arriving on the scene will be encountering an unknown, potentially hostile environment, where one or more combatants may have been, and possibly still are, armed. Like any sane person, they will be concerned, cautious, and likely at least a little bit scared. Since they do not know exactly what transpired, they also do not know yet who the good guy is and who the bad guy is.

A confrontational attitude will do you no good and may well guarantee that you will be arrested or shot. Several undercover officers have been killed by their uniformed counterparts when they failed to follow directions immediately and/or did not identify themselves properly. If you are training a weapon on a subdued attacker, be sure to follow the responding officer's instructions immediately, without any hesitation. While the officer does not know whether you are the good guy, he knows with absolute certainty that you are armed and dangerous. You don't want to survive a violent confrontation only to be killed afterward due to a preventable misunderstanding.

Be respectful, courteous, obedient, and kind, but remember that the officer(s) is/are not your friend. The officer's job is to secure the environment, provide for first aid, gather facts, and enforce the law. Consequently, he will not necessarily be on your side no matter how prudently you acted, at least not until all the facts are known.

Control your emotions to the extent possible. Carefully and calmly, explain what happened so that the responding officer(s) will know that you are the good guy. Retain your composure and conduct yourself in a mature manner, avoiding any words or actions that may appear threatening or volatile. Police are trained interrogators. They will note your body language, speech patterns, and eye movements to help ascertain your probable guilt or innocence when deciding whether to make an arrest. And they will err on the side of caution, so even a suspicion of guilt may be enough to earn you a night in jail.

Say as little as possible. Do not, under any circumstances, make any incriminating statements that may be used against you at a later time. Do not confess to any crime, even if you think you exercised poor judgment or are guilty. Here is an example of something you might say that is perfectly honest and should be relatively well received:

> "This was a very traumatic experience. I think I'm in shock.
> I don't think I should say anything until I'm calmer. Can I
> please call [your attorney or contact person]?"

Officers usually distinguish between a debrief/interview conducted at the police station, where legal representation is appropriate, and a tactical debrief that takes place at the scene. If you withhold information that endangers officers, you will not make friends and could get someone seriously hurt, but information you give could (rarely but theoretically) incriminate you.

While there may be a fine balance between implying guilt through silence and being overly talkative, err on the side of caution. You do not have to say anything at all without an attorney present, though it is generally prudent to identify yourself and state that the other person attacked you and that you were in imminent and unavoidable danger, fearing for your life. You may even wish to explain why you could not simply run away. If you used a weapon and have a concealed weapons permit, it is generally a good idea to let the officers know that as well.

Be polite and respectful to the jail guards too. They can deny you phone access and generally make your life even more miserable if you act inappropriately. In most jurisdictions, you must be taken before an officer of the court (e.g., judge, magistrate) within twenty-four hours of your arrest, except on weekends. You should always secure counsel and have legal representation before this initial court appearance. If you cannot afford an attorney, you can be represented by a public defender, though that is not ideal.

CHAPTER FIFTEEN

Legal Matters

Police Officers Don't Like Fighting, So They Don't Like You

The fight is over, the police have arrived, and somebody is going to jail. Responding officers really don't care a whole lot about how it started or what you were fighting about. A couple of questions to make an assessment, and more often than not somebody gets arrested. Judges and juries determine guilt or innocence; officers eliminate the immediate threat and control the danger that you and/or your adversary caused to the public.

You might think that what you are involved in is the most important thing in the world at that moment. You might be fighting over the love of your life, defending your honor, trying to get paid for a bet or a loan, or collecting something that was stolen from you. It might be very important to you, yet these officers have just left a scene just like yours to deal with you. And the odds are good that they'll get another half dozen calls just like yours before the night is over.

From the jaded perspective of a veteran officer, you're really not that special. You're barely a name, let alone a face. Your story,

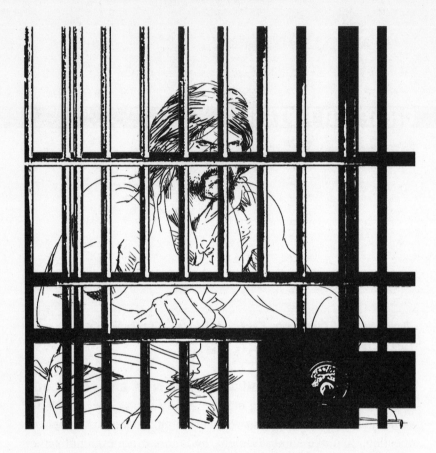

your issues, they mean absolutely nothing to these guys. The officers cannot afford to get emotionally involved; they have a job to do. Now, don't take that as an anti-cop comment, because it is not. They have a dirty, unglamorous, rotten job to do that few are willing to take. We should all be damned thankful that there are people willing to step up and do it. The challenge is that in order to survive on the mean streets of most any city, a certain level of emotional detachment has to come with the territory.

Officers have to have a shell; without it, they can't function. They are not bad people, they just see, hear, and feel too much to allow an emotional attachment for every person and every problem. You with your petty problems don't have a chance of cracking that shell.

Find a Good Attorney

If you've been in a fight, there is a good chance that you'll be charged with a crime. And you're woefully unprepared to defend yourself in court. That's like a weekend golfer trying to compete with Tiger Woods. You could get in a lucky shot and win a hole or two, but your odds of victory over an eighteen-hole course are minuscule.

You need the best attorney (or team of attorneys) you can afford to help you out. The legal fight is just as dangerous if not more so than the physical fight you survived. Lose this one and you may very well lose your freedom, your job, your house, your relationships, and your money. Relying on an underpaid, overworked public defender appointed by the court is the last thing you should do unless you have no other choice.

It is useful to have an attorney in mind before you need one. It's downright imperative if you have a concealed weapon permit and carry a firearm or work in a violence-prone vocation (e.g., bouncer, bounty hunter, security guard). The challenge is that surfing the Net or browsing the yellow pages is a time-consuming, haphazard way to find one. A good place to find a solid reference is through a friend or relative. Even if they have only used someone for civil matters such as creating a will, their attorney will likely know someone who specializes in criminal defense law. If you are enrolled in college, you can check with the law school there. They will often have an excellent referral service. You can also contact the bar association where you live or work to find someone.

You need a lawyer who has a long track record in the applicable field of law, someone who has successfully worked on cases like yours. For example, a DUI attorney might be the top player in his field, a real expert at defending accused drunk drivers, yet totally incompetent to handle a murder case.

Since many violent crime cases are settled with a plea bargain instead of going to trial, you will want someone who has experience adjudicating a case like yours through the whole process.

If you are innocent, pleading guilty to a lesser offense would be highly inadvisable in most instances.

In firms with multiple attorneys, different lawyers may handle different cases or different aspects of the same case. Be sure to meet the person who will be representing you. If a team is likely to be involved, be sure to meet with each specialist before agreeing to anything. This reasonable request should be accommodated. You are the paying customer; it's your welfare on the line.

Ascertain how reliable, available, and responsive your prospective lawyer is likely to be. Most attorneys keep a running backlog of cases, managing multiple clients at the same time. Regardless, it is important that you be able to contact your attorney whenever you need assistance throughout the legal process as well as whenever any new information about your case may arise. You may be relying on this person not only to defend you in a criminal court but also in any follow-on civil procedure as well, so you don't want someone who's too busy to give you his or her best work.

Once you have selected someone to defend you, you will need to be patient and cooperate. Never forget that your attorney is your lifeline, protecting your freedom and reputation. While you are bound to be anxious and generally afraid, the justice system moves rather slowly at times.

Ask about the costs, benefits, and risks of pursuing any particular legal strategy. Cooperate with your defense attorney to help expedite the process. Be willing to do some of your own legwork, gathering documents and information as requested. Keep a log of any questions you might have so that you can discuss them during regular consultations rather than contacting your attorney every time something pops into your head.

As your case progresses, your attorney will work with you to develop a plan for securing your freedom and restoring your reputation. Criminal defense strategies can include alibis, justifications, procedural defenses, and excuses. While the particulars of each case will be different, alibis and justifications are fairly common and are generally effective defense strategies. Procedural and excuse defenses can be challenging to prove in a court of law. There are a few other innovative defenses as well, but they are unorthodox, fairly rare, and not generally effective.

■ An alibi is based upon the premise that you are completely innocent and can prove that you were in another place when the alleged act was committed, so you could therefore not possibly be guilty.

■ A justification is a claim that, while you admit that you committed the act, you should not be held liable for your actions because of certain special or extenuating circumstances. A justification for murder, for example, is a legitimate claim of self-defense (which makes it not a murder in the eyes of the court).

■ A procedural defense attempts to prove that while you broke the law, you cannot be held criminally liable because the state violated a procedural rule. Examples include entrapment, prosecutorial misconduct, double jeopardy, or denial of a speedy trial. In these instances, you may have done something wrong but cannot be found guilty.

■ An excuse is an argument that you were not liable for your actions at the time a law was broken. Examples include diminished capacity, duress, or insanity. While you may not be criminally liable in such instances, you may still be civilly committed to professional counseling to ensure that you recover from the illness that let you off the hook.

■ Other so-called innovative defenses can include allegations of long-term abuse, battered women's syndrome, urban survival syndrome, and other creative things that lawyers occasionally use to try to convince a jury to acquit a defendant. These things rarely work, however, and are generally not something a prudent attorney would try. Be cautious if your attorney suggests pursuing this line of defense.

Realize That Courts Are About Resolution, Not Justice

If you are looking for justice from the courts, you are playing a fool's game. Courts are not interested in justice, they are interested in resolution. While judges are honorable, hardworking individuals, the courts are jam-packed with cases and notoriously understaffed—in some areas, they're completely overwhelmed. Courts are designed to process people and come to resolution. Justice is an expensive commodity. The police do their job and the courts do theirs. Unfortunately, if you engage in violence, you will get pinched in the middle.

Look at the lists of people with rap sheets five feet long who are still out on the streets—these guys became professional criminals a long time ago. If there was justice, they wouldn't be out preying on the weak, vulnerable, aged, and defenseless of our society. Jail to these professional criminals means three free meals a day, long showers, plenty of sleep, and a great opportunity to study up on what they did wrong and refine their technique. It is a nice respite to help them get ready for their next go in the world of violence and crime.

Facing a shortage of bed space, severe overcrowding, and a lack of taxpayer willingness or political wherewithal to build additional facilities, prisons throughout the country are forced to make tough decisions. They use a variety of processes to identify low-risk offenders to routinely release prisoners early. Unfortunately, there is rarely such a thing as "low risk" when it comes to criminal offenders.

According to the Bureau of Justice Statistics, recidivism rates are very high. About 3 percent of the adult population has spent time in prison. That's not jail, mind you, but prison, the place where you are sent for serious crimes with convictions that result in long-term sentences. Jail, on the other hand, is where inmates are locked up for a relatively short time, such as those awaiting trial or serving a short-term sentence. Almost three-quarters of parolees are rearrested for felonies or serious misdemeanor crimes within three years of release. About half of those are reconvicted for a new crime.

You, most likely, are not a professional criminal. That means that you are just the kind of person the justice system likes. You are inclined to make bail (that costs you money). You are likely to show up in court with an attorney (that costs too). You are looking to earn some sort of parole (that takes time, and time equals money). Depending on what you have been accused of, you might well be assigned a psychiatric examination (that costs money) and a violence education program (that takes a lot of time, the cost for which you have the privilege of paying too).

In short, as a regular, generally law-abiding citizen, you are also an easy mark for the courts. You will bear the full brunt of the legal system. You can pad their conviction statistics by pleading guilty to a lesser crime in order to avoid the risk of an extended prison stay. In most cases, you probably shouldn't cop a plea, but you certainly may be tempted to. After all, you value your life and your lifestyle. The professional criminal, on the other hand, couldn't care less what the judge says. The threat of a jail stay or prison term is not an earth-shattering, life-changing event as it would be to the rest of us. It is, rather, a minor inconvenience.

We've all seen examples in the news where celebrities who can afford handlers, fixers, and small armies of attorneys can get away with things that the average citizen cannot. Despite the tabloids and the headlines, however, the justice system really does work pretty well much of the time. Even the rich and famous can wind up doing hard time when they get caught. Imagine how much worse it might be for you, the not so rich and mostly anonymous.

Your best bet is keeping your nose clean, but if you ever do find yourself caught up in the legal system, it is paramount that you have an excellent attorney to help you navigate the process. It's expensive, time-consuming, and fraught with peril. Think about that the next time you're in the mood to hit someone.

CHAPTER SIXTEEN

You've Got a "Stay Out of Jail Free" Card If You Use It Wisely

Countervailing force, or physical self-defense, is vio-lence applied against an aggressor to keep him from hurting you. In the process, you may intentionally or unintentionally injure, maim, cripple, or even kill your adversary. If you only give the other guy a bloody nose or a minor bruise, it can still have serious repercussions, such as a night in jail or a nice, fat, juicy lawsuit. Because of this possibility, it is important to understand how your actions might be scrutinized under the law.

A legitimate case of self-defense and a good lawyer can get you off the hook most, but not all, of the time. Consequently, it is really important to know when you're on solid legal ground. We're martial artists, not attorneys, so nothing in this book constitutes a legal opinion, nor should any of its contents be treated as such. The law is very nuanced, so talk to a qualified lawyer to understand the specifics of laws in your jurisdiction.

The AOJP Principle

The AOJP principle is a good way to ascertain whether it makes sense to use physical force in a self-defense situation. AOJP stands for Ability, Opportunity, Jeopardy, and Preclusion. If all four of these criteria are met, you have a pretty good legal case for taking action.

Ability

Ability means that an attacker has both the physical as well as practical ability to seriously injure, maim, or kill you. This may include the use of fists and feet as well as the application of conventional or improvised weapons such as knives, guns, bottles, baseball bats, or similar instruments. It also includes the physical ability to wield said weapon (or fists or feet, for that matter) in a manner that can actually injure you. A small child with a baseball bat does not have the same ability to cause you harm as a professional ballplayer swinging the same hunk of wood as a weapon. Similarly, unless there is a massive skill differential, a petite woman has less ability to hurt you with a punch or kick than a muscular man.

Opportunity

While your attacker may have the ability to harm you, his ability does not necessarily mean that he also has the immediate opportunity to do so. Your life and well-being must be in clear and present danger before you can legally respond with physical force. For example, a bad guy with a knife has the ability to kill you only so long as he is also within the striking range of the weapon or can quickly move into the appropriate distance from which to initiate his attack. A physical barrier such as a chain-link fence may protect you from a knife wielder but not from an assailant armed with a gun, so opportunity relates not only to the attacker and the weapon but also to the environment within which they are deployed.

Jeopardy

Jeopardy, or "imminent jeopardy" as the law sometimes requires, relates to the specifics of the situation. Any reasonable person in a similar situation should feel in fear for his life. This is a legal attempt to distinguish between a truly hazardous situation and one that is only potentially dangerous. While you are not expected to be able to read an aggressor's mind, you certainly should be able to ascertain his intent from his outward appearance, demeanor, and actions. Someone shouting, "I'm going to kill you," while walking away is probably not an immediate threat even though he may very well come back later with a weapon or a group of friends and become one if you stick around long enough. Someone shouting, "I love you," while lunging toward you with a knife, on the other hand, most likely is an imminent threat.

Preclusion

Even when the ability, opportunity, and jeopardy criteria are satisfied, safe alternatives other than physical force must be precluded before you can legally engage an opponent in combat. If you can run or retreat from harm's way without further endangering yourself, it isn't necessary for you to use violence. In some jurisdictions, there is no requirement to retreat when attacked in your home or, in some cases, your place of business. Regardless, it is prudent to retreat whenever you have the ability to do so safely. After all, it is impossible for the other guy to hurt you if you're not there.

If all four of these criteria are met, you have a pretty good legal case for taking action. If one or more of these conditions is absent, however, you are on shaky legal ground.

Conclusion

> I cleansed the mirror
> of my heart—now it reflects
> the moon.
> —RENSEKI (1701-1789)[6]

Violence is a complex and disturbing subject, one that requires careful study and firsthand experience to truly understand. In this book, we have presented what we hope is a clear, thorough, realistic, and thought-provoking analysis of violence. You have read real-life examples of violent people, examined their brutal behavior, and have a good understanding of the harsh realities of the aftermath of violence.

Now that you have finished the book, you should be able to recognize behaviors, both in others and in yourself, that may lead to a fight. Understanding these situations can help you make the right choices for success in conflict resolution. Sometimes you really do need to fight, yet most of the time it's the wrong thing to do.

To summarize what you've read, we would like to leave you with these four simple rules of self-defense:

■ **Rule Number One:** Don't get hit. That's primarily about using awareness, avoidance, and de-escalation to eliminate the need to fight in the first place. Where a physical confrontation is unavoidable, it's also about warding off the other guy's blows so that you can counterattack successfully.

■ **Rule Number Two:** Stop him from continuing to attack you. A purely defensive response is insufficient in a street fight, as it can only keep you safe for a very short period of time. You must stop the assault that is in progress so that you can escape to safety or otherwise remain safe until help arrives. Your goal is to be safe, not to kill your attacker or teach him a lesson.

■ **Rule Number Three:** Always have a Plan B. No matter how good a fighter you are, whatever you try is not necessarily going to work. The other guy will be doing his damnedest to pound your face in, pulling out every dirty trick he can think of in an effort to mess you up. It is prudent, therefore, to have a Plan B, some alternative you can move to without missing a beat when things go awry.

■ **Rule Number Four:** Don't go to jail. This is about judicious use of force, knowing when it is appropriate to take action as well as knowing how much force to apply. The AOJP principle can hold you in good stead during conflict situations.

Now is the right time to put some heavy thought into what you have learned. Flip back to the "How Far Am I Willing to Go?" checklist. See if what you have read changes any of your original answers.

Be smart, use your head, and stay safe.

Endnotes

1. Sunao (1887–1926) was a haiku poet. This was his death poem, written shortly before he died at the age of thirty-nine. Haiku is a traditional epigrammatic Japanese poem based on seventeen syllables that are arranged in three lines, five syllables in the first and last lines and seven syllables in the second line. Translation from the original Japanese reads:

> Spitting blood   chi o hakeba
> clears up reality   utsutsu mo yume mo
> and dream alike   saekaeru

2. Togyu (1705–1749) was a haiku poet. He died on August 15, 1749, at the age of forty-four. Translation of his death poem from the original Japanese reads:

> When autumn winds blow   Nan no mama
> not one leaf remains   nokoru ha mo nashi
> the way it was   aki no kaze

3. Sosen (1694–1776) was a haiku poet. He died on June 28, 1776, at the age of eighty-two. Translation of his death poem from the original Japanese reads:

> Lotus seeds   Hasu no mi no
> jump every which way   tobitokoro arı
> as they wish   shinjizai

4. Ryushi (1684–1764) was a haiku poet. He died on September 6, 1764, at the age of seventy. Translation of his death poem from the original Japanese reads:

Man is Buddha— *Mi wa hotoke*
the day and I *ware to iu hi wa*
grow dark as one *kurenikeri*

5. *Miranda v. Arizona*, 384 U.S. 436. Ernesto Miranda was arrested for robbery, kidnapping, and rape in 1963. He was subsequently interrogated by police and confessed to his crimes. Prosecutors offered only his confession as evidence during his trial, where he was convicted. The Supreme Court later ruled in 1966 that Miranda was intimidated by the interrogation, understanding neither his right to not incriminate himself nor his right to have counsel present during the interrogation. On the basis of that finding, the court overturned his conviction. He was later convicted in a new trial where witnesses testified against him and other evidence was presented, and served eleven years for his crimes. This Supreme Court ruling forms the basis of the "Miranda Rights" that all suspects must be read prior to interrogation by law enforcement.

The actual wording states,

The person in custody must, prior to interrogation, be clearly informed that he has the right to remain silent, and that anything he says will be used against him in court; he must be clearly informed that he has the right to consult with a lawyer and to have the lawyer with him during interrogation, and that, if he is indigent, a lawyer will be appointed to represent him.

Police are only required to Mirandize an individual whom they intend to subject to custodial interrogation. While arrests can occur without questioning and without the Miranda warning, the warning must be given prior to any formal interrogation.

6. Renseki (1701–1789) was a haiku poet. He died on July 5, 1789, at the age of eighty-eight. Translation of his death poem from the original Japanese reads:

I cleansed the mirror *Harai aria*
of my heart—now it reflects *kokoro no tsuki no*
the moon *kagami kana*

Bibliography

Books

Artwohl, Dr. Alexis, and Loren W. Christensen. *Deadly Force Encounters: What Cops Need to Know to Mentally and Physically Prepare for and Survive a Gunfight.* Boulder, CO: Paladin Enterprises, Inc., 1997.

Ayoob, Massad F. *In the Gravest Extreme: The Role of the Firearm in Personal Protection.* Concord, NH: Police Bookshelf, 1980.

———. *The Truth About Self-Protection.* New York: Bantam Books (Police Bookshelf), 1983.

Christensen, Loren W. *Far Beyond Defensive Tactics: Advanced Concepts, Techniques, Drills, and Tricks for Cops on the Street.* Boulder, CO: Paladin Enterprises, Inc., 1998.

———. *Gangbangers: Understanding the Deadly Minds of America's Street Gangs.* Boulder, CO: Paladin Enterprises, Inc., 1999.

———. *Riot: A Behind-the-Barricades Tour of Mobs, Riot Cops, and the Chaos of Crowd Violence.* Boulder, CO: Paladin Enterprises, Inc., 2008.

———. *Surviving Workplace Violence: What to Do Before a Violent Incident, What to Do When the Violence Explodes*. Boulder, CO: Paladin Enterprises, Inc., 2005.

Consterdine, Peter. *Fit to Fight: The Manual of Intense Training for Combat*. Chichester, UK: Summersdale Publishers, 1998.

———. *Streetwise: The Complete Manual of Security and Self Defence*. Chichester, UK: Summersdale Publishers, 1998.

———. *Travelsafe: The Complete Guide to Travel Security*. Leeds, UK: Protection Publications, 2001.

De Becker, Gavin. *The Gift of Fear and Other Survival Signals That Protect Us from Violence*. New York: Dell Publishing, 1998.

Grossman, Dave, and Loren W. Christensen. *On Combat: The Psychology and Physiology of Deadly Conflict in War and Peace*. Belleville, IL: PPCT Research Publications, 2004.

Hoffman, Yoel. *Japanese Death Poems: Written by Zen Monks and Haiku Poets on the Verge of Death*. Rutland, VT: Tuttle Publishing, 1986.

Kane, Lawrence A. *Surviving Armed Assaults: A Martial Artist's Guide to Weapons, Street Violence, and Countervailing Force*. Boston: YMAA, 2006.

Kane, Lawrence A., and Kris Wilder. *The Way of Kata: A Comprehensive Guide to Deciphering Martial Applications*. Boston: YMAA Publication Center, 2005.

———. *The Way to Black Belt: A Comprehensive Guide to Rapid, Rock-Solid Results*. Wolfeboro, NH: YMAA Publication Center, 2007.

Luttrell, Marcus, and Patrick Robinson. *Lone Survivor: The Eyewitness Account of Operation Redwing and the Lost Heroes of SEAL Team 10*. New York: Hachette Book Group, 2007.

MacYoung, Marc. *A Professional's Guide to Ending Violence Quickly*. Boulder, CO: Paladin Enterprises, Inc., 1993.

———. *Cheap Shots, Ambushes, and Other Lessons: A Down and Dirty Book on Streetfighting and Survival*. Boulder, CO: Paladin Enterprises, Inc., 1989.

———. *Fists, Wits, and a Wicked Right: Surviving on the Wild Side of the Street*. Boulder, CO: Paladin Enterprises, Inc., 1991.

———. *Floor Fighting: Stompings, Maimings, and Other Things to Avoid When a Fight Goes to the Ground.* Boulder, CO: Paladin Enterprises, Inc., 1993.

———. *Knives, Knife Fighting, and Related Hassles: How to Survive a Real Knife Fight.* Boulder, CO: Paladin Enterprises, Inc., 1990.

———. *Pool Cues, Beer Bottles, and Baseball Bats: Animal's Guide to Improvised Weapons for Self-Defense and Survival.* Boulder, CO: Paladin Enterprises, Inc., 1990.

———. *Street E & E: Evading, Escaping, and Other Ways to Save Your Ass When Things Get Ugly.* Boulder, CO: Paladin Enterprises, Inc., 1993.

———. *Taking It to the Street: Making Your Martial Art Street Effective.* Boulder, CO: Paladin Enterprises, Inc., 1999.

———. *Violence, Blunders, and Fractured Jaws: Advanced Awareness Techniques and Street Etiquette.* Boulder, CO: Paladin Enterprises, Inc., 1992.

Miller, Rory. *Meditations on Violence: A Comparison of Martial Arts Training and Real World Violence.* Wolfeboro, NH: YMAA Publication Center, 2008.

Morgan, Forrest E. *Living the Martial Way.* Fort Lee, NJ: Barricade Books, Inc., 1992.

Musashi, Miyamoto. *A Book of Five Rings: The Classic Guide to Strategy,* trans. Victor Harris. Woodstock, NY: The Overlook Press, 1974.

Quinn, Peyton. A *Bouncer's Guide to Barroom Brawling: Dealing with the Sucker Puncher, Streetfighter, and Ambusher.* Boulder, CO: Paladin Enterprises, Inc., 1990.

———. *Real Fighting: Adrenaline Stress Conditioning Through Scenario-Based Training.* Boulder, CO: Paladin Enterprises, Inc., 1996.

Rapaport, Samuel. *Tales and Maxims from the Midrash.* London: George Routledge & Sons Limited, 1907. Available at www.sacred-texts.com/jud/tmm/index.htm.

Sde-Or (Lichtenfeld), Imi, and Eyal Yanilov. *Krav Maga: How to Defend Yourself Against Armed Assault.* Tel Aviv: Dekel Publishing House, 2001.

Sutrisno, Tristan, and Marc MacYoung. *Becoming a Complete Martial Artist: Error Detection in Self-Defense and the Martial Arts.* Guilford, CT: The Lyons Press, 2005.

BIBLIOGRAPHY

Tzu, Sun. *The Art of War*. Text only, no commentary, trans. Lionel Giles. Project Gutenberg eBook, December 28, 2005 (eBook #17405).

Articles

Ayoob, Massad. "One Gun, No Hands: The Marcus Young Incident." (The Ayoob Files) *American Handgunner*, September–October 2004.

DVDs and Videos

Barroom Brawling: The Art of Staying Alive in Beer Joints, Biker Bars, and Other Fun Places (with Peyton Quinn and Marc MacYoung). Paladin Press, 1991.

Street Safe: How to Avoid Becoming a Victim (with Marc MacYoung). LOTI Group Productions, 2007.

Street Smarts: How to Avoid Being a Victim (with Detective J. J. Bittenbinder). Video Publishing House, Inc., 1992.

Web Sites

Bureau of Justice Statistics: www.ojp.usdoj.gov/bjs

Crime Check: www.crimecheck.com

Federal Bureau of Investigation Uniform Crime Reports: www.fbi.gov/about-us/cjis/ucr

In the Line of Duty: www.lineofduty.com

No Nonsense Self-Defense (Marc "Animal" MacYoung's Web site): www.nononsenseselfdefense.com

Net Detective: www.netdetective.com

Seattle Post-Intelligencer: www.seattlepi.com

Sentry Link: www.sentrylink.com

The Art of War: www.chinapage.com/sunzi-e.html

BIBLIOGRAPHY

A Book of Five Rings: www.samurai.com/5rings

Mayo Clinic: www.mayoclinic.com

The Seattle Times: www.seattletimes.nwsource.com

U.S. Search: www.ussearch.com

Yahoo! News: news.yahoo.com

About the Authors

Kris Wilder

Having begun his martial arts training in 1976 in the art of tae kwon do, Kris Wilder has earned black-belt-level ranks in three arts: tae kwon do (second degree), Kodokan judo (first degree), and Goju Ryu karate (fifth degree), which he teaches at the West Seattle Karate Academy. He has trained under Kenji Yamada, who as a judoka won back-to-back United States grand championships (1954 and 1955); Shihan John Roseberry, founder of Shorei-Shobukan karate and a direct student of Seikichi Toguchi; and Hiroo Ito, a student of Shihan Kori Hisataka (Kudaka in the Okinawan dialect), the founder of Shorinji-Ryu Kenkokan karate.

Now retired from judo competition, while active in the sport Kris competed on the national and international levels. He has traveled to Japan and Okinawa to train in karate. He is the author of *The Way of Sanchin Kata* and *Lessons from the Dojo Floor* and coauthor (with Lawrence Kane) of *The Way of Kata, The Way to Black Belt,* and *The Little Black Book of Violence*. He has also written guest chapters for other martial arts authors and has had articles published in *Traditional Karate,* a UK magazine with international readership. Kris regularly instructs at seminars internationally. Kris is a University of New Mexico Institute of Traditional Martial Arts National Representative.

Kris lives in Seattle, Washington, with his son, Jackson. He can be contacted via e-mail at kwilder@quidnunc.net or through the West Seattle Karate Academy Web site at www.westseattlekarate.com.

Lawrence Kane

Lawrence Kane is the author of *Surviving Armed Assaults, Martial Arts Instruction,* and *Blinded by the Night,* as well as coauthor (with Kris Wilder) of *The Way of Kata, The Way to Black Belt,* and *The Little Black Book of Violence*. He also has published numerous articles about teaching, martial arts, self-defense, and related topics; has contributed to other authors' books; and acts as a forum moderator at www.iainabernethy.com, a Web site devoted to traditional martial arts and self-protection. Lawrence is a technical consultant to the Institute of Traditional Martial Arts at the University of New Mexico.

Since 1970, he has participated in a broad range of martial arts, from traditional Asian sports such as judo, *arnis, kobudo,* and karate to re-creating medieval European combat with real armor and rattan (wood) weapons. He has taught medieval weapons forms since 1994 and Goju Ryu karate since 2002. He has also completed seminars in modern gun safety, marksmanship, handgun retention, and knife combat techniques, and he has participated in slow-fire pistol and pin shooting competitions.

Since 1985, Lawrence has supervised employees who provide security and oversee fan safety during college and professional football games at a Pac-10 stadium. This part-time job has given him a unique opportunity to appreciate violence in a myriad of forms. Along with his crew, he has witnessed, interceded in, and stopped or prevented hundreds of fights, experiencing all manner of aggressive behaviors as well as the escalation process that invariably precedes them. He has also worked closely with the campus police and state patrol officers who are assigned to the stadium and has had ample opportunities to examine their crowd-control tactics and procedures.

To pay the bills, he does IT sourcing strategy and benchmarking work for an aerospace company in Seattle, where he gets to play with billions of dollars of other people's money and make really important decisions. Lawrence lives in Seattle, Washington, with his wife, Julie, and his son, Joey. He can be contacted via e-mail at lakane@ix.netcom.com.